By the same author
ANTIQUES OF THE PHARMACY

THE ANTIQUES
OF PERFUME

Leslie G. Matthews

LONDON : G. BELL & SONS: 1973

© LESLIE G. MATTHEWS 1973
PUBLISHED BY G. BELL & SONS LTD
YORK HOUSE, 6 PORTUGAL STREET, LONDON WC2A 2HL

PRINTED IN GREAT BRITAIN BY
W & J MACKAY LIMITED, CHATHAM

ISBN 0 7135 1756 5

Contents

List of Plates

Following page 20

Following page 76

NOTE

Numbers in parentheses in the text refer to Plates

Acknowledgments

In the preparation of this book I have had much help from The Director, Archives de la Seine, Paris; The Director, Archives Nationales de Paris; Monsieur D. Beutlung, Les Parfums Worth, Paris; Miss Valerie Bartlett, The Beauty Centre, London; The Director, Bibliothèque Historique de la Ville de Paris; Mlle Antoinette Boisguilbert, Attachée de Presse, Bourgois, Paris; Henry Brocksom, Esq., London; Dr J. K. Crellin, Wellcome Institute of the History of Medicine, London; Madame Galby, Roger & Gallet, Paris; Madame Gaudin, Archiviste, Bouvet Collection, Paris; Mrs E. C. Hannam & G. V. J. Budd, Esq., J. & E. Atkinson Ltd, London; Mr W. H. Helfand, Paris; Monsieur Henri Jeanjan, Les Cristalleries de Baccarat, Paris; J. L. Howgego, Esq., Keeper of Prints & Pictures, Guildhall Museum, London; Miss Judith Holmes, Public Relations, Coty, London; Madame Lagouet, Syndicat National des Fabricants de Produits Aromatiques de Synthèse, Paris; Miss Lydia Mez-Mangold, Curator, Schweizerisches Pharmaziehistorisches Museum, Basle; Monsieur Pierre Migeot, Givaudan S. A., Paris; Miss E. Morgan, Asprey & Company, London; The Librarian and Staff of the Library of the Pharmaceutical Society of Great Britain, London; The Librarian, Reckitt and Colman, Ltd, Hull; Monsieur Martin Schneider, F. Hoffmann-La Roche & Co., Basle; Mlle Francoise Soubrette, Attachée de Presse, Syndicat National de la Parfumerie Francaise, Paris; Miss Olive Stephens, Public Relations, International Perfumery Centre of Proprietary Perfumes Ltd, Ashford, Kent; Madame Monette Wolber, Agence de Presse, Les Parfums Chanel, Paris; and Miss Adrienne S. Wood, Houbigant Inc., Ridgefield, New Jersey, USA.

In Grasse I benefitted from discussions with a number of perfumers, including Monsieur Jose Aime, Lautier Fils; Monsieur Paul Giampetro, Directeur des Relations Exterieurs, Parfumerie Fragonard; Monsieur H. Honnerat, Molinard and Bertrand Frères. I should mention particularly the kindness of the Pharmachim State Economic Trust, Sofia, who through the Bulgarian Trade Commissioner, London, supplied me with literature and photographs relating to the Bulgarian perfume industry. The editors of the *Chemist & Druggist* and the *Pharmaceutical Journal* have readily allowed me to reproduce matter published in their respective journals.

ILLUSTRATIONS I should also like to record my thanks to those who have kindly provided photographs and other material as illustrations and who retain the copyright in them:

Asprey & Company, London, Nos. 7, 10, 43

Bearnes & Waycott, Torquay, No. 56

Gerard Bryant, Esq., London, No. 83

The Conseil d'Administration de l'Ordre des Pharmaciens, Paris, Nos. 78a, 80a, 80b, 87

Christie, Manson & Woods, London, Nos. 29, 30

The Curator, Cromwell Museum, Huntingdon, Nos. 25, 27

Coty, London, No. 14

Eric Delieb, Esq., London, No. 32

Givaudan S.A., Vernier-Geneve, Nos. 8, 39, 41, 42, 46, 47, 48, 49, 57

The Government of India Tourist Office, London, No. 4

George B. Griffenhagen, Washington, U.S.A., Nos. 65, 81, 86, 88

Guerlain, Parfumeurs, Paris, Nos. 17, 20, 69, 75

The Director, Guildhall Museum, London, Nos. 84, 85

Houbigant Inc., Ridgefield, New Jersey, U.S.A., No. 60

Mrs. G. E. P. How, London, No. 31

F. Hoffmann-La Roche & Co. Basle, Nos. 1, 9, 35

The Director, The London Museum, Nos. 11, 51, 52, 58, 76, 79a, 79b

Miss Margaret Medley, Curator, Percival David Foundation of Chinese Art, London, No. 3

A. & F. Pears, Ltd, London, No. 89

M. le Directeur, Musée Périgord, Périgueux, No. 77

Parfumerie Fragonard, Grasse, No. 67

P. S. Peberdy, Esq., Curator, Southampton, Museums, Nos. 33, 34

The Pharmaceutical Society of Great Britain, Nos. 16, 61, 62, 63, 70, 74

Pharmachim State Economic Trust, Sofia, Bulgaria, Nos. 19, 21, 22, 23, 24

Marcus Samuel, Esq., London, No. 12

Dr C. H. Spiers, No. 55

Sotheby & Co., London, No. 66

G. R. A. Short, Esq., No. 18

The Trustees of the British Museum, No. 5

The Victoria & Albert Museum, No. 50

The Wellcome Trust, London, Nos. 2, 6, 13, 26, 28, 36, 37, 38, 40, 44, 45, 53, 54, 59, 64, 68, 72, 73

The House of Yardley, London, Nos. 15, 71

L.G.M.

Introduction

Most plants and flowers have a characteristic odour, not always pleasant but in the main agreeable. Scenes and people are often recalled by an aroma associated with them and when names are forgotten the scent of a particular perfume can bring back memories. 'L'odorat est le sens du souvenir.' According to Rudyard Kipling, each country has its own odour: this was true of all the countries he had visited. Another writer, Eugène Fromentin, was reputed to have such a remarkable sense of odours that he could tell by the odour whether he was at the Pole or the Equator.

The art of perfumes has been described as the most evocative for each of the senses—subtil, profound and penetrating, the art of silence, at once provocative and soothing. Whereas music disperses, perfume concentrates the attention.

The rapid growth of the perfumery industry during the nineteenth century mirrors the rise of the middle classes whose wealth grew as their manufactories increased in importance. Madame de Staël once attributed the birth of the modern perfumery industry in the mid-nineteenth century as issuing from 'la mode, de la chimie, et du commerce', all three developments coming at the one time. The identification of odours from natural sources and the synthesis of compounds having similar or slightly different properties enabled the perfumers to add to their range of materials and so produce new perfumes having what is called a new 'note' or attractiveness, increasing the variety offered to the public. In this the 'nose' of the perfumer is all-important. A keen sense of odour can be cultivated, but like the blender of brandies or wines, the perfumer does best if he is born with that indefinable sense that enables him to appreciate the value of a trace of this or that ingredient which can make all the difference to a new production.

The present century has seen an eruption of new perfumery houses, catering for every size of purse. No longer are the mudpacks of Southend needed to cleanse and beautify the complexion. Cosmetic creams intended to maintain or renew youthful looks have appeared in variety as never before, some medicated with hormones, radioactive substances or dyes, in addition to those designed to effect weight reduction. Whereas formerly men tended to regard the use of perfume as effeminate, in recent years special perfumes have been created for them and use of these is growing.

When perfumes were a luxury and so within the reach of only the wealthy, the containers, the flacons and scent bottles had to be works of art distinctive of their period. In the eighteenth century therefore we find richly-chased gold containers embellished with enamels and decorated by artists of the highest repute. Important collections of these are now in private hands or not infrequently have been gathered by owners of some of the leading perfumery houses such as Fragonard, Givaudan, Guerlain, Houbigant and Ed. Pinaud, to mention only a few.

While choice containers like scent bottles were the objects associated with perfume that chiefly attracted collectors during the past hundred years, the present-day collector may feel disposed to include perfume and cosmetic cases, porcelain and pottery jars or even labels to increase the variety and interest in his chosen subject. Under the heading 'Some Collectable Antiques' (Chapter 6) the reader will find descriptions of many objects additional to those discussed in other chapters of this book.

I

The Perfumes of Ancient Peoples

O F the ancient peoples whose use of perfumes, aromatic oils, unguents and cosmetics has been recorded, none have left better remains than the Egyptians, the Greeks and the Hebrews. Not only are the names and kinds of ingredients given but there is good evidence of the specific use of the compounds, with descriptions of the containers in which they were stored.

The Egyptians

In Egypt aromatic gums and woods were regularly burned by the Priests in the Temple of Isis. On special occasions the King himself would take part in the ceremonies, censer in hand, or would pour wine or perfumed oils as libations. On feast days, the body of an ox would be filled with myrrh and other aromatics to counteract the unpleasant smell of the burning of the sacrificial beast. Rameses III (XIX dynasty), in an invocation to the god Ammon, when asking for some service of the god, exclaimed: 'Have I not sacrificed 3,000 oxen, with all the accompanying aromatic herbs and the choicest perfumes?'

At Heliopolis incense composed of several ingredients, including resins and myrrh, was offered to the Sun God at sunrise, midday and sunset. Vases of alabaster, many of which were engraved, contained the fragrant ointments forming part of the offerings. Aromatic pastilles were burnt in the sacred lamps.

The Egyptians set the fashion, later adopted by the Greeks and Romans, for the use of aromatic oils after bathing. These oils were kept in special vases or boxes, some in the form of ducks or fishes. Many workers were engaged in preparing a variety of cosmetics. There was a green eye-paint made from soot, burnt almond shells or galena (lead sulphide), with

[1]

malachite, a green carbonate of copper, to which was added a resin from conifers; and lip colouring prepared with fats and floral perfumes or aromatic resins, the floral perfumes being extracted by a process of *enfleurage* described on page 46. Pomades in balls or cones were often worn on the head.

The first bottles for perfumes were made in terracotta and only much later in glass, though glass techniques were being developed during the 4th millenium BC. By the middle of the second millenium a complicated process of glass bottle-making involved winding molten glass round a shaped core of sand and clay, the neck being constricted by coloured threads; finally hot glass threads in many colours were wound round the bottle, which when combed gave coloured striations, vertical or wavy. For perfumed ointments, squat decorated jars were preferred. Surviving terracotta bottles, especially those of the late sixth century BC made as grotesque heads or sphinx-like, suggest the use of moulds or of considerable skill in direct embellishment before firing.

In the Greek Islands Egyptian influence led to the production of similar types of perfume bottles. For example, in Cyprus poppy-head bottles have been discovered, dated to about 1500 BC, scarred in imitation of the scarring of the poppy capsules when opium was to be obtained from them.

Some museum specimens of Egyptian alabaster containers of the second millenium BC, used for eye make-up and for ointments and oils, bear such names as Pharaoh Amenophis, Queen Teje and Queen Hatsheput (*c.* 1375 to 1350 BC).(1) Kohl, a black antimony powder for darkening the eyelids, was applied with a fine pencil-like bodkin, and a lady's toilet case would usually contain red and white paints to heighten the complexion. Fingers and palms of the hand were stained with henna, the powdered leaf of a herb, *Lawsonia alba*, or the fingers might be gilded. For driving away wrinkles of the face a recipe lists balls of incense, wax, fresh oil and cypress berries, all crushed, rubbed down and put into new milk, the mixture to be applied to the face for six days.[1] Illustrations show the use of mirrors and of wooden combs. Wigs were commonly used by the well-to-do. When a guest arrived his wig or shaven head would be anointed with perfumed oils.

A further important use of aromatic substances such as myrrh and

---

[1] Wootton, A. C., *Chronicles of Pharmacy*, London, 1910, *I*, 44, quoting from Budge, A. W., *Guide to the Egyptian Collection in the British Museum*, London, 1909, 34.

cassia was for embalming. These substances, with bitumen, were injected or inserted into the body of the cadaver when the intestines, etc., had been removed. The body could then be sewn up, and kept in natron, a kind of soda plentiful in Egypt, for a period, after which it was wrapped in layers of linen and deposited in a wooden case. Highly decorated mummy cases are the prize exhibits of many museums. The viscera, heart, lungs, liver and gall were carefully preserved in funeral vessels called 'canopic jars'. The house could be purified with 'kyphi', a sacred perfume composed of myrrh, juniper berries, frankincense, perfumed woods and other ingredients.

Baldness was a trouble to the Egyptians as long ago as 1550 BC. In one of their medical treatises, the *Papyrus Ebers*, discovered by George Ebers and named after him, written about that time, are two formulae to make the hair grow. Neither would commend itself today. One contained oil of the Nile horse, with mint, myrrh and the like; the other called for the heels of the greyhound and of asses to be boiled in oil with date blossoms. To prevent the hair turning grey, either the fat of a rattlesnake or the blood of a black calf was to be boiled in oil and applied to the scalp.[2] Amongst the Romans the nearest preparation of this kind of thing was the plentiful use of pomades, and in nineteenth-century England, the well-advertised bear's grease.

Greece

Perfumes played a great part in Greek life. Most of the classic authors refer to their use, as offerings to the Gods,[3] in everyday life in the home, to provide fragrance in cooking, and for personal enjoyment. Perfumes were also used in the treatment of the sick and some, like rosewater, were employed for diseases of the eye. The Greeks recognized the special virtues of the essences and oils from the East. Three classes of traders were well established: the *arômatopôlès*, sellers of aromatics, the *myrépsos*, purifiers of myrrh, and the *muropôlès*, the myrrh sellers.

Greek perfume containers were made in a variety of substances, among them onyx and alabaster, many being exquisitely carved. A particular

---

[2] Wootton, *op. cit.*, I, 42.

[3] 'Celestial Venus hover'd o'er his head And roseate unguents heavenly fragrance shed' (Iliad).

type of archaic Corinthian terracotta vessel round in shape with flattened head, about 8 cm. high, called *aryballos*, was common in the early sixth century BC. These vases, for perfumed unguents, are often found decorated with rosettes and rows of padded dancers or with figures in black whose eyes are recessed to show the clay colour underneath.(2) Scent bottles were made in the shape of animals' heads or women's heads from the classical type to the everyday peasant.

The Greeks knew that when perfume was applied to the warm hand its fragrance was intensified. At banquets therefore it was necessary for youths to present to each guest sweet and costly perfumes before the meal. The perfumes themselves were prepared by steeping flowers in oil. The aromatic unguents contained powders from roots and gums. Greek vases depict all aspects of daily life, including scenes of ladies at their toilet.

The Hebrews

The practices of the Hebrews in the small Kingdoms of Israel and Judah regarding sacrificial offerings and the use of oils and unguents for anointing purposes appear to have been much like those of Egypt and the inhabitants of their neighbouring territories, save that for the most part in their religious observances they were monotheistic. Now and again however, according to their prophetic books, they had to be warned of the error of adopting the gods of their neighbours. To what degree the books of the Pentateuch are truly representative of the history of the Hebrews is a matter for debate but the details of their practices in using incense and of anointing their kings as a seal and acceptance of a chosen leader, are clearly set down. Thus, Aaron was to burn sweet incense every morning and Moses was to make 'an oil of holy ointment' of pure myrrh,[4] sweet cinnamon, sweet calamus, cassia and olive oil, 'after the art of the apothecary' (or perfumer),* for anointing Aaron and his sons, to be used only for this purpose. Sweet spices too, were to be pounded to make a perfume

---

[4] Myrrh was used profusely. *The Song of Solomon* (4, 5) refers to 'mountains of myrrh and the hill of frankincense'.

* In modern Israel the Hebrew name for a pharmacy is BETH MIRKACHAT (The House of Mixing) and the two words ROKEACH (pharmacist) and MIRKACHAT (to mix or to distil perfume) are from the same root. (Michaels, I. *Pharm. Jnl.*, 1971, *207*, 137.)

'after the art of the perfumer', to be regarded as most holy (Exodus 30, 34–7). Saul, the first King of Israel, was anointed with a phial of oil by Samuel (1 Sam. 10). Asa, King of Israel, was buried in a bed or tomb filled with sweet odours and divers kinds of spices prepared by the apothecary's art (2 Chron. 16).

The Talmud, largely completed between 500 and 200 BC, gave specific directions for the preparation of a temple incense, based upon the Exodus formula, to which was added a herb to cause the smoke to ascend straight. Many other passages in the Old Testament and in the Apocryphal Books mention the art of the apothecary or perfumer.

The Jewish practice of anointing the head with a sweet-smelling pomade or unguent evidently continued into the early part of our era, to judge by the account of the woman who had an 'alabaster box of very precious ointment' for this purpose (Matthew 26), and the bringing of sweet spices for anointing to a sepulchre as was done by the three women was also customary (Mark 16).

Personal adornment amongst the Hebrews, including the use of kohl for darkening the eyes, was well known and the subject of unfavourable Biblical comment from time to time. That this practice has continued in Palestine through the centuries is exemplified in a recent exhibition arranged by the British Museum, where a Galilee tribeswoman's garments included her kohl bag, trimmed with feathers, coins and tassels, evidently a prized possession.

The Balm of Gilead, often mentioned, appears to be a sweet gum-resin, probably from small trees grown in the Gilead area. The name was in use by many quack medicine exponents in the eighteenth century and later for a general heal-all.

The Romans

If the early Romans adapted Etruscan ideas of living, they borrowed equally from the Greeks, particularly in the field of medicine. Rome itself was doctored by Greek physicians who either came willingly or as vanquished in the wars. The luxurious habits of the Greeks commended themselves to their Roman masters. During the centuries of the Republic, before 27 BC, the lavish use of perfumes had already begun. This increased under the Empire. The arts of the *unguentarius*, maker of pomades, and the *myropolae*, perfumers and sellers of balsams, flourished. In the time of the Emperor Augustus the perfume called 'Rhodinium', made from the roses of Paestum, was so highly prized that it sold for its weight in gold. Public baths were built by emperors—those of Caracalla are still one of the sights of Rome—and they became the fashionable meeting places for the exchange of gossip and for intrigues. After bathing, scraping and massage, the bodies of the bathers were anointed with perfumed oils or pomades, rose or narcissus being greatly favoured. Whatever they fancied to use in their homes—perfumes or pomades in bottles or jars of glass or alabaster—could be readily purchased. So lavish was their use that Martial in one of his epigrams castigates a young lady smothered in perfume, saying that his dog, if so treated, would smell every bit as well as she.

The Roman ladies had no need to follow Ovid's recipes for beautifying themselves: there were plenty of face washes, pastes and creams for the complexion and preparations for darkening the eyes. Among those regularly used was Galen's Cold Cream, *crema* or *unguentum infrigidans*. Galen, celebrated Græco-Roman physician and pharmacist of the second century AD, born in Pergamon of Greek parentage, wrote innumerable books on all facets of disease, on the restorative and ameliorative uses of massage and on the virtues of medicated oils. He was an authority on this subject, having been at one period physician to a group of gladiators. His famous Cold Cream was made by melting white wax in olive oil in which rose buds had been macerated. The mixture, poured frequently from vessel to vessel, with cold water stirred in, became white. A general formula based upon Galen's was in use for centuries, and, though modified many times, Cold Cream has remained on sale longer than any other beautifier. Glazed earthenware pots, with decorated lids bearing the name of the maker, were in use as containers for it into this century.

China

For centuries incense has been burnt on the altars of temples. In later periods, for example in the seventeenth century, cylindrical wide-mouthed jars were used as receptacles for it. They can be found decorated in blue, sometimes with dragons, and may be inscribed with verses indicating the dedication of the vessel as a perpetual offering in the Hall of the Three Religions—Confucianism, Buddhism and Taoism.

Clothes were kept sweet with scented powders. Pomades for the hair contained musk, patchouli, sandal, ambergris and asafetida. Asafetida, though much used in India as an aromatic condiment, has never become popular in Europe, even when employed as a medicine in cases of hysteria, because of its penetrating persistent odour.

The usual method of perfuming rooms has been to burn joss sticks that give off a pungent smell. The name 'joss' is said to be a corruption of the Portuguese 'dios' (God). The use of gilded perfumed papers ('batonets' in French), was considered indispensable for banquets at the beginning of this century. Rose petals, jasmin flowers and chrysanthemum leaves were employed to add fragrance to tea leaves: the presentation of such highly perfumed tea was regarded as a gracious offering to a friend.

Although there are many thousands of beautifully carved Chinese snuff bottles of all periods in jade, semi-precious stones, crystal, agate, lacquer, etc., it is rare indeed to find a Chinese perfume bottle, though some snuff bottles without the inserted needle or spoon may be mistaken for perfume bottles. Perfume cups are equally rare. A fascinating cup of the Ming period, late sixteenth century, displayed in the Percival David Foundation of Chinese Art, London, takes the form of a whole lichee and a half lichee, part glazed, part in biscuit, with a perforation where the two fruits meet so that the perfume could run from one to the other. It was apparently intended to perfume a room or to be used at table.(3)

Arabia

From time immemorial Arabia has been known for its production of spices and gums, the bases of so many perfume materials used in ancient times. For centuries it had a widespread trade, both for its indigenous output and its commerce with India and the Far East. It is not surprising therefore that the Arabs themselves should have cultivated the habit of using perfumes. Musk was one of their favourites. The Koran notes the use of musk, called the seal of musk, and mentions too, damsels with dark eyes. Thompson[5] repeats the traditional story that two mosques, Tauros and Kara Amed, had musk incorporated in the mortar when they were being built, so that in the warm sunshine the whole buildings would give

[5] Thompson, C. J. S., *The Mystery & Lure of Perfume*, London, 1927, 32.

off an agreeable aroma. The Arabs' use of perfume in cooking is well attested.

It was the Arabs who from the ninth century developed science and utilized the full knowledge of the time. One of the achievements of Arab pharmacists was the distillation of rose water in the eighth century though crude methods for this are mentioned as early as the second century BC by Nicander, a writer on medical and pharmaceutical practice.*

India

India has always been regarded as a country in which the use of perfumes flourished. The religious ceremonies of both Hindu and Muslim communities demanded the offering of incense and of this sandalwood and gums, products of the country, have been the main ingredients. Coffrets of the sandalwood of Mysore were for long treated as cult objects. Today a mixture of powdered sandalwood, gums and resins is used to coat small bamboo sticks for burning. These are termed 'Mysore agarbathis'.

Attars, the distillate of flowers have always been produced in India; of these rose and jasmine are the two most important. In former times attars were made by primitive methods: a small alembic was encased in a kiln of brick; a spout of bamboo protruding from the alembic served as a condenser. The essence of sandal, for example, was heated over a fire with water and jasmine flowers were dropped into the hot oil which was then distilled. Second and third additions of jasmine flowers allowed an added concentration of the final product. This was very precious.

To make snuffs, tonka beans and synthetic essences are added to the ground tobacco. Cedar and sandalwood soaps represent a considerable part of the output of the Mysore factories.

Make-up has not been neglected by Indian ladies: eyelid shadow powder and eyelash darkener were, and are, part of the everyday materials

---

* Holmyard gives details of a rudimentary apparatus for distilling found at Tape Gavra in the north-east of Mesopotamia, dating from about 3500 BC. By means of a double-lidded pot, the lower lid channelled for holding a concentrated liquid, the vapour from the bottom of the apparatus could be condensed into the liquid which then ran back for re-distillation. The chemist of today terms this 'reflux distillation.' (Holmyard, E. J., *Alchemy*, Harmondsworth, 1957, 42.)

for heightening the lustre of the eyes. Make-up boxes are still given as wedding presents by bridgegrooms.

Besides its own perfumes, India offers to the collector a choice of many objects resulting from the age-old handicrafts.(4) Painted clay vessels, metal wares such as powder boxes in brass or copper repoussé work, in which the design is hammered from the reverse side, and powder boxes in lac are made in great variety. Bidri wares, first made in Bidar, now almost the only place where this kind of work is carried on, first came into prominence in this country during the eighteenth century. These wares have their designs in silver or gold on black metal. Indian enamel work includes the making of globular, long-necked rosewater sprinklers, the designs on which make these a fascinating study.

2

Medieval to Elizabeth I

IT was not until the return of those Crusaders who had enjoyed the unexpected luxurious kind of life they found in the East that the use of
perfumes became general in Western Europe, though St Médard had
established the Crown of Roses in the sixth century and paladins of the
Court of Charlemagne (d. 814) returning from the East had reported on
the use of perfumes there. There is occasional mention of kings and
nobles during the Anglo-Saxon period making use of perfume and by the
tenth century aromatic unguents and perfumes were known generally
throughout the whole of the Mediterranean basin. All efforts to suppress
this by legislation were in vain.

In France there was official recognition of perfumers by Philip Augustus in 1190 and in 1268 the Corporation of Maistres Gantiers (Master
Glovers) was formed. From the very beginning they sold an assortment of
perfumes, hair dyes and cosmetics. For some centuries the preparation
and sale of these was mainly in their hands. This is not to say that the
Glovers had it all their own way: the Merciers or Haberdashers acted on
the principle that what the Glovers sold they too could sell and the
rivalry between them was acute. In 1594 neither body was allowed to
nominate its members as perfumers but in 1614 the Glovers succeeded in
securing the right to do so and this was confirmed in 1691 and held good
until the Revolution of 1793 which put an end to this monopoly. Up to
that time a would-be perfumer served a four-year apprenticeship, three
years as an assistant, and was then designated a master-perfumer.

In Court circles in both France and England apothecaries were often
called upon to provide sweet smelling substances for their royal masters
and their wives. Some of the accounts of Odinet the spicer for medicines
supplied to Isabella, daughter of Philip IV of France and wife of Edward II,
included perfumes. Odinet had probably been engaged by Isabella during
her visit to France in 1312. He charged for roseated oil, made by macerat-
ing rose petals with roses and camomile, or roses, violets and camomile, in

olive oil. He also furnished incense (frankincense) to perfume her rooms, in addition to damask rose water and violet flowers.[1]

During Edward II's reign Robert the Spycer supplied ambergris, billed as 'ambre', in the form of a comforting electuary, a sweet jam-like conserve containing ambergris, musk, pearls, jacinth, gold and silver. Rose sugar was obviously much appreciated by most monarchs of that period; surviving bills record many supplies of this. Whilst King John of France was held hostage in Somerton Castle, Lincolnshire, in 1359, his own apothecary who had come over from France, made for him and his retinue, comfits or dragées of rose-flavoured sugar and conserve of rose and damask rose.[2]

Even if bathing was not regularly practised by royalty in the fifteenth and sixteenth centuries, at least the monarchs saw to it that their clothes and bed linen were cleaned. The officers of the Wardrobe of Edward IV (d. 1483) had instructions for washing and cleansing the royal apparel, and the King's robes, doublets, sheets and shirts had to be 'fumed' throughout the year by the yeoman apothecary. This was considered so important that the Chamberlain had to record when it was done. The grooms and pages had orders to gather sweet flowers, herbs and roots to make the King's gowns and sheets 'brethe more wholesomely and delectable'.[3] All this was in keeping with Edward's known propensity for the company of pretty women. Edward's daughter, Elizabeth, later the wife of Henry VII, followed her father's style: she had bags or sachets perfumed with orris and anise.[4] Sachets had become popular after the Glovers of France began to make them, then called 'coussins', filling them with rose and lavender.

Thomas Norton of Bristol who in 1477 had drawn attention to the value of smell in detecting changes in the preparation of chemicals refers to the use of sweet smelling substances in his day: 'Pleasant Odours ingendered be shall Of cleane and Pure substance and fumigale, As it appeareth in Amber, Narde and Mirrhe, Good for a Woman, such things pleaseth her'.[5](5)

---

[1] Trease, G. E., The Spicers and Apothecaries of the Royal Household . . ., Hen. III, Ed. I, E. II. *Nottingham Medieval Studies*, 1959, III, 19–52.

[2] Matthews, Leslie G., 'King John of France and the English Spicers', *Medical History*, 1961, V, 65–76.

[3] Myers, A. R., *The Household of Edward IV*, Manchester Univ. Press, 1959, 117–20.

[4] *Liber Niger Domis Regis Angliae Ed. IV. Harl.*, 642, 131, 137, 147.

[5] *The Ordinall of Alchemy*, in which he wrote: 'Smelling maie helpe forthe your intente, To know your reigning Elemente'. Facsimile reproduction, London, 1928.

Catherine of Medici on her marriage to Henri II of France in 1533 not only brought her Florentine cooks with her, which in the view of many changed the character of French gastronomy,[6] but also her own perfumer. He was allowed to set up a shop on the Pont au Change in Paris and his customers increased in number rapidly. At a later period, 1548, the City of Paris decided to have the waters of public fountains perfumed with aromatic herbs and plants.[7] There is no record of this having been repeated. The public have preferred the fountains to run with wine, as they did in London on special occasions, rather than with pleasantly flavoured waters.

Stimulated by the increase in knowledge of natural substances, new inventions and better laboratory equipment, there grew up towards the end of the sixteenth century a new type of professional, the chemist, distinguished from the apothecary whose main interest was in the sale of drugs and the preparation of medicines. These new men familiarized themselves with the art of distillation not only for their novel chemicals but in order to make all kinds of distilled waters, essences and perfumes. Hieronymous Braunschweig had published his book on the distillation of herbs, *Liber de Arte distillandi* in 1500 and an English version was printed by Laurence Andrew, London, in 1527.

It was doubtless following the new knowledge that the distilling of sweet waters during the reign of Henry VIII became customary. The plentiful use of these by the monarch himself and his Court provided almost a full time occupation for the royal yeoman apothecary. In 1529 no fewer than twenty-seven waters were distilled, including damask rose, red rose, rosemary, bean flower, honeysuckle and scabious. Besides there were listed some twenty-four 'Old waters of the last year remaining', mostly of flowers, broom, eglantine, marigold and yarrow.[8] Some of these waters could have been added as flavourings to sauces and jellies or sweetmeats.

Though it has been said that perfumes did not come into general use in England until the reign of Queen Elizabeth I (1558–1603),[9] this cannot

---

[6] Oliver, Raymond, *The French at Table*, The Wine and Food Society, London, 1967.

[7] Rimmel, Eugène, *The Book of Perfumes*, London, 1865, 200.

[8] British Museum MS Royal 7c xvi, fos. 98–99.

[9] Rimmel, Eugène. *Op. cit.* Rimmel quotes from Howes that it was Edward de Vere, Earl of Oxford, who first brought perfumed gloves, sweet bags, a perfumed leather jacket and other pleasant things from Italy. Elizabeth was so pleased to be

be so for poets and playwrights were so often mentioning them. In the *Winter's Tale*, Act IV, sc. iv, Autolycus offers: 'Gloves sweet as damask roses; Masks for faces and for noses; Bugle bracelet, necklace amber, Perfume for a lady's chamber.' The use of bellows to provide a sweet smelling atmosphere—the 'Fresh-air' aerosols of the seventeenth century —were noted by John Ford: 'I'll breathe as gently as a perfumed pair of sucking bellows in some sweet lady's chamber.' In France, Cardinal Richelieu is reported to have employed bellows regularly to perfume his apartments. Certainly Henry VIII's apothecaries and perfumers were well able to prepare perfumes for that monarch himself and for the Court. A recipe of one of his perfumers included compound water, cloves, rose water, fine sugar, musk, ambergris and civet. So highly aromatic was this that the instructions were to 'boil it gently together' otherwise all the house would smell of cloves.[10] Henry VIII was also supplied with pastille burners, called 'fuming boxes'.

The account rendered by Thomas Alsop, the King's chief apothecary during the last months of the King's reign, 1546–7, records many supplies for royal use.[11] Wherever he was in residence, at Oatlands, Nonsuch, Sheen or Windsor, there was perfume for the King's use and for the Chamber; a box with fine perfumes for the Admiral of France, a half-gallon silver flagon of rosewater, and several frontals (face masks) of sandal. The apothecary's duties included the preparation of the King's bath with bags of herbs, sponges, musk, civet and spices; no doubt intended to give relief to the King who was then suffering badly with dropsy and swollen legs. One of the King's Court singers, Mr Hylle, had a box of cold cream, noted as Infrigerans Gallen. For Princess Mary, later Queen Mary, there were quantities of sweet waters made with rosemary and lavender. She also had sweet bags filled with crushed orris root, rose leaves and aromatic gums. Perfume was sent to her at Windsor for her chamber.[12] King Edward VI had perfume to make his house 'smell like rose water'.

The most informative account we have of the use of perfumes at the

presented with perfumed gloves that she wore them for several of her portraits, having at the same time a girdle strung with pomanders.

[10] *Privy Purse Expenses of Henry VIII, 1529–32*, Ed. N. H. Nicolas, London, 1827, 232.

[11] *Letters & Papers of Henry VIII*, Vol. XXI, pt. 2, 394–9.

[12] *Privy Purse Expenses of Princess Mary, 1536–64*. Ed. F. Madden, London, 1831, 74–8.

Court of Queen Elizabeth I is the detailed bill of John Hemingwey, appointed apothecary to the Queen in 1558. He had been a yeoman apothecary to Henry VIII but does not appear to have served Queen Mary. The bill for the first six months of 1564, January to June,[13] shows with what regularity perfumes for all kinds of purposes were needed. This was the year when the Queen started to dress her hair in a new style, wearing a wig because she was losing her own hair rapidly.

Every two or three days Hemingwey supplied perfume, rosewater and cloves for the 'Closetts', the cupboards or presses in which clothes were kept. Benjamin and storax, sweet smelling gums, were sent for the robes and rosewater, a pint or more at a time. The robes worn were so heavy, often fur-lined and so much bedecked with jewels, that perfuming them was the only way of keeping them sweet. Then there was perfume for the chapel, usually an ounce at a time, for the council chamber, and for the great chamber. Pounds of orris root, violet powder, were sent to the Ladies of the Bedchamber to see that the linen was perfumed, and now and then damask powder. Comfits, sweetmeats, or sugar plums were scented with musk. When the Queen was carried in a litter, perfume for this was required, and again for the gallery in which she stood for her public appearances.

The Queen would have everything sweet smelling about her, and like her father, had her special bath scented with herbs and spices. This was done about once a month. The bath may have been enclosed so that the bather sat upon a padded board to have the benefit of the aromatic fumes. When the Queen visited Windsor the bath was taken there. The Queen took pains over her complexion. Her apothecary had to provide face masks by making a cold cream, spreading this upon parchment which was then covered with sarcenet, a fine soft silk material, and quilted. This was applied at night.

Not only did she insist upon having her own rooms well perfumed[14] but when there was a visit of importance from M. de Gonnor, the French Ambassador, she gave instructions that his lodgings at Sheen had to be perfumed before his arrival and the Banquetting House similarly treated when he was to be present.

---

[13] British Museum MS. Sloane 5017*.

[14] In 1960 the Laboratories of The Wellcome Foundation, London prepared for Queen Elizabeth the Queen Mother a quantity of a room fumigant made to an ancient recipe which was a favourite of Queen Elizabeth I. (*Pharm. Journal*, 1960, *185*, 502.)

The Queen delighted in receiving presents and her physician, Dr Robert Huycke, always remembered this. One of the gifts he made her at the New Year was of toilet waters, a square perfuming pan of silver plate and a pomander 'garnished with gold and twelve sparks of rubies'. There was still a need for pomanders, regarded as effective in warding off plague.[15]

From the fourteenth to the seventeenth centuries there were constant exhortations to avoid infection from all pestilential airs. Some plague tracts recommended purifying the air by disinfection, others like that of Sir John de Mandeville, 1365, additionally advised carrying a pomander in the hand. The use of 'pommes' or 'barillets', small cylinders, containing strong perfumes to prevent the plague is recorded of the Dukes of Normandy in the fourteenth century. It was claimed that heavily-scented materials comforted the brain and gave protection against any miasma or airborne disease. An inventory taken at the death of Charles V in 1380 shows that he possessed various pommes ambres, embellished with precious stones, pearls and other costly jewels.

The pomander was a mixture of aromatic substances in which were included musk, civet and ambergris (the last-named then known as 'ambre', hence the name pomme ambre), to provide a pleasant smell and to mask the odour of some of the other ingredients. Carrying a pomander in the hand was not always convenient and small chains were added to the containers to allow them to be hung from the belt, suspended from the neck or attached to the purse that hung down from the girdle. Monumental effigies showing balls resembling oranges attached to the wrists or suspended from the belt are not uncommon. Cardinal Wolsey was a firm believer in simply perfumed pomanders: several of his portraits show him holding a spiced orange to his nose.

At the height of the Great Plague of 1665 the College of Physicians of London was asked to suggest remedies and to give preventive advice. A list of ingredients was published and the apothecaries had the remunerative task of putting them into a mass, sold at twelve pence each, suitable for whatever kind of container the customer might choose. Most of these containers were perforated to permit the sniffing of the contents whenever the holder felt himself in danger. People in high places, the monarch,

---

[15] Two wills of Bury St Edmunds, Suffolk, record legacies of gold pomanders: Agnes Hals, 1554, 'My pomander of gold', and John Baret, 1643, 'Item, to my Lady Walgrave my musk ball of gold with purple and lace'. (*Wills and Inventories . . . Commissars of Bury St. Edmunds*, etc. Ed. Samuel Tymms, *Camden. Soc.* 1850, 49.)

nobles and the gentry, sought to have their pomanders in gold or silver decorated with precious stones in fanciful designs suggested by the gold-smiths and jewellers.

Silver pomanders were sometimes made with folding leaves enclosing orange-like segments, the whole resembling an apple when closed. The segments containing the aromatic substances, rose, mace, caraway and similar ingredients, might have the names engraved upon them, perhaps for convenience when refills were needed.(6) Pomanders in the form of spinning tops, the upper rounded portion also containing a vinaigrette, might be closed with a silver thimble, large enough to hold a nutmeg. (13, right) All sorts of shapes were made; globular, apple, pear, are only a few of the many examples, varying in height to about 8 cm.(13, left) The less wealthy had to make do with a wooden pierced ball opening into two halves.

Stick pomanders were customary at the end of the sixteenth century and some of the gold-headed canes carried by physicians, almost as a badge of rank, had a cavity in the head with a screw or lift-off top into which a pomander could be inserted. The idea that sweet aromas could ward off infection or harmful and noxious odours has been kept alive, though perhaps with no real conviction, in the custom of the posies of flowers carried by H.M. Judges in the Courts and by the Lord Mayor and Aldermen in the City of London on special occasions. As soon as vinai-grettes became popular in the early part of the eighteenth century pom-anders fell into disfavour.

3

The Stuart Period to the End of the Eighteenth Century

COURT life changed quickly once James I succeeded Elizabeth I in 1603. Places had to be found for James's Scottish followers. A new Lord Chamberlain was appointed with complete control of the household staff, many of whom procured their places by purchase. The customary gifts to the monarch at New Year by members of his staff continued, his two physicians offering pots of green ginger and orange flowers.

Though in some respects James I has the reputation of boorishness, nevertheless he dressed well, at least his portraits suggest this, he loved jewellery, and, judging by the bills submitted by his apothecary, Joliffe Lownes, for the three months from April to July, 1622, he saw to it that his person and his rooms were well perfumed. The King was supplied with sweet powder for his teeth and with orange flower water and rose water. Powder and rose water were sent to his barber; his personal and table linen had to be scented and when he went from St James's to Theobalds, Greenwich or Richmond, quantities of perfume were sent beforehand to the grooms who were to prepare his rooms. Even the King's barge and his coach had to be perfumed, a commentary upon the malodorous state either of the barge-master and the crew or the coachman.[1] No wonder that John Wolfgang Rummler, a foreigner, and apothecary to both James I and his Queen, and whose duties included supplying sweet powders and perfumes, could submit a bill in 1610 for these things amounting to almost £800.

Queen Henrietta Maria who was married to Charles I in 1625 brought with her a number of Ladies, Demoiselles and Officers who were to be her personal servants in England. Amongst them were an apothecary and a perfumer, Jean Baptiste Ferione. Nevertheless one of Charles's apothe-

---

[1] *Proc. Soc. Antiq.*, London, Sec. Ser. IV, 435–7.

caries still retained the duty of supplying sweet waters to the royal Family. It was about this period that the fashion of wearing perfumed gloves had taken a firm hold amongst the nobility. In 1622 the Countess of Pembroke ordered no less than 99 pairs of gloves at a time from Lesgu, a Paris haberdasher. They were to be scented with orange flower water or ambergris.

Ben Johnson, in *The Silent Woman*, written about 1600, Act. IV, Sc. 1, had already given the current view on women's make-up: Truewit, talking of the Lady Haughty, says: 'Women ought to repair the losses time and years have made in their features with dressings. And an intelligent woman, if she know by herself the least defect, will be most curious to hide it; and it becomes her'.

Although after 1618 the Apothecaries had claimed the sole right of making distilled waters, the London distillers, whose members were chiefly concerned with strong liquors and vinegars, contested this. The Distillers' Company was incorporated in 1638 on the strong representations made by Sir Theodore Turquet de Mayerne and Dr Cadman. They gained the right to distill all those waters which were not in the London Pharmacopoeia or were not prescribed by physicians.

Once Charles II was firmly on the throne in 1660, life at Court took on a new freedom. Forgotten was the earlier Puritan condemnation of worldly adornment. Charles had already made up his mind in what style he would live and it was soon apparent that in habits and dress his reign would outdo his predecessors. Long curled wigs for men and decolleté dresses for the ladies were quickly adopted. For the King's own head there were bags of perfumed powder, and for his wardrobes and the chapel similar bags, with perfumes for the Privy Galleries and the royal apartments; these, with sweet waters for the royal household were ordered from his apothecary.

Sweet bags, i.e. large sachets to hold perfumed powder, were so much in demand for the linen of the King and Queen Catherine that each year, beginning in 1661, 24 yards of crimson taffeta, 20 sets of fine holland, and 24 crimson galloons, silk laid, were issued so that the apothecary could have the requisite bags made. When the Court was at its most sumptuous, the use of patches and powder was at its height. Ladies' dress and their complexions had to be seen in daylight and by candlelight. For the less favoured, recipes of all kinds were published and quack vendors guaranteed dazzling complexions by the use of their washes and pastes. Some of these, containing mercury, were positively dangerous, as was the Duchess of

Newcastle's recommendation in her *Poems & Fancies* to use a strong sul-phuric acid to remove the outer layer of skin, to induce a more blooming complexion underneath. Every artifice was practised to enhance beauty and to exhibit it. The great period of Lely as portrait painter had arrived, to be followed by Kneller.

Another well-tried means of achieving a good complexion was to bathe the face in May dew. For this the early morning on the first day of May was considered best. Mrs Pepys, to the annoyance of her husband, went out early more than once to get the May dew. Many ladies tried it but the benefits are unrecorded. If they needed warrant for the practice they could find it in the writings of William Salmon, an inveterate publicist on medical matters in the second half of the seventeenth century.[2] 'May dew', he wrote, 'exceeds all others for purity, clarity, penetration and volatility.' He even suggested the distillation of May dew, with the object of producing 'Spirit of Rain'.

Of the use of patches, first adopted by the Court ladies of France, early in the seventeenth century, we have news of the custom in the Hague on 14 May 1660 when Samuel Pepys, riding in a coach with Mr Creed and two pretty ladies, notes they were 'very fashionable and with black patches'. It was not long before the fashion spread to London, for on 31 August of the same year, the Diarist writes: 'This the first day that ever I saw my wife wear black patches'.[3] At first the patches were small but they began to be cut into diamond, star and crescent shape, even as a coach and horses and face and breast were decorated with them.

Despite the increased demand for perfumery of all kinds, stimulated by the Court of Charles II, perfumers seem to have had no guild or organization of their own, the usual practice of groups of artisans or pro-fessionals who had their own Companies or Guilds in London and in most cities and large towns. During Charles II's reign when Huguenots of all trades and professions fled to Britain from France and the Low Countries, many of whom remained in London, only a handful of them are recorded as *parfumeurs*.

Thomas Shadwell, writing his satire on the Royal Society and on scientific collecting in *The Virtuoso*, published 1676, lists most of the perfumer's stock-in-trade: this included gloves, amber, orangery, frangi-

[2] Salmon, W., *Pharmacopoeia Londinensis*, London, 1691, 4th ed. 437.
[3] Latham, R. and Matthews, W., *The Diary of Samuel Pepys*, London, 1970, I, 138, 234.

pane, neroly, tuberose, jessamin (jasmine), Marshall,* washes, pomatums,†
and confections to restore the complexion. John Jackson, Samuel Pepys's
younger nephew, on a visit to Rome for the Holy Year, sent his uncle
from Leghorn on 18/29 July 1700 a box containing amongst other items:
2 small boxes of Florentine essences, 2 ivory boxes of Roman apopletick
balsam, a Frenchpan ball, a small paper of pastilles to burn, and several
pairs of Roman gloves, some perfumed with double franchpane, neroli,
castor or jasmine and six pairs of gloves 'in walnut shells, Roman', in
addition to 3 pots of Naples soap and 3 lb. Venice treacle.[4] ('The gloves
packed in walnut shells were probably of the thinnest kind, made of
chicken skin.)

It was during the last years of Charles II's reign that the wars with
Louis XIV cut off supplies of French perfumes and cosmetics. These then
had to come in from Italy. Shipments through Amsterdam in 1684 included casks of Hungary Water, hair powder, perfume bags and jasmine
oil. There was still a considerable risk of plague. Several severe outbreaks
were noted and preventives were strongly recommended, such as those in
A Rich Closet of Physical Secrets,[5] in which it was suggested windows should
be decked out with flowers, carnations, roses and herbs, and the floors
should be strewn with rushes, oak and willow leaves, and mints. A sweet-
scented bag ought to be worn over the heart,(9) a pomander, nodule or
nosegay carried in the hand, and, in an infected area, a piece of angelica
root, citron peel or cloves should be held in the mouth. The nodules
described were to be made of flowers, coarsely powdered, tied into a
piece of taffeta and wetted with rosewater and vinegar before smelling
them.

The practice of strewing herbs in churches and in the Guildhall,
London, goes back for centuries. At the Court of Hustings, when the Lord
Mayor and the Sheriffs of the City of London are elected each year on 29
September, the end of the Guildhall should be sprinkled with aromatic

---

* A powder attributed to Madame la Marishale d'Aumont, wife of Antoine,
Mareshal de France, d. 1669.

† Pomatum (Pomade). This denoted a soft smooth paste with a texture somewhat
like cold cream. The name was first applied in 1637 by Jean de Renou to a medicinal
ointment containing apples (pommes), hence the term 'pomade' and only later came
into general use for all kinds of semi-solid creamy preparations for external use.

[4] Pepys, S., *Private Correspondence & Misc. Papers, 1679–1703*, Ed. J. R. Tanner,
London, 1926.

[5] Printed by Gartrude Dawson, London, 1652.

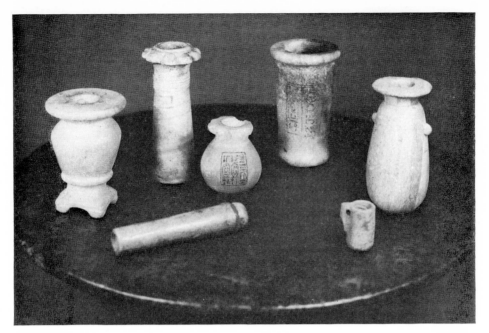

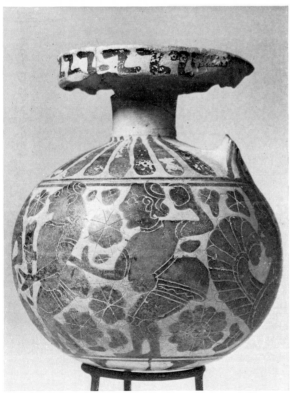

1. (above) CONTAINERS FOR COSMETICS, 2ND MILLEN-IUM B.C.

Left to right: Egyptian alabaster vase for Kohl. Height 7.5 cm. Egyptian alabaster tube, palm column. Height 9.5 cm. Egyptian alabaster pot bearing the names Pharaoh Amenophis and Queen Teje. Height 4.5 cm. Egyptian alabaster pot bearing the name Queen Hatshe-put. Height 8 cm. Greek alabaster pot for ointments or perfume. Height 8 cm. Foreground: Kohl tube, blue faience, Egyptian, Height 8 cm. Egyptian Perfume bottle, blue-green faience. 3 cm. (From A History of Drugs *by Lydia Mez-Mangold)*

2. ARYBALLOS—PERFUME CONTAINER, CORIN-THIAN, c. 600 B.C.

Decorated with padded dancers and siren, left. Five dancers have red faces, one a black face. Height 8 cm. (Wellcome Institute of the History of Medicine)

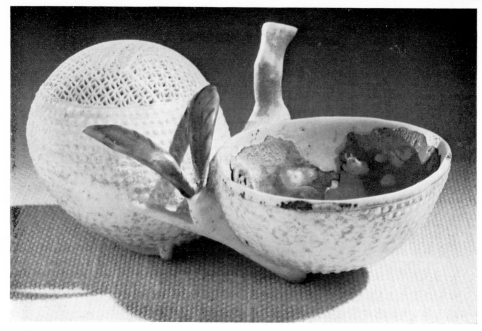

3. *(above)* CHINESE PERFUME CUP, MING, LATE 16TH CENTURY
In the form of a lichee and a half lichee. Blue and white with poetic inscription in open-work. Width 12.1 cm. (Percival David Foundation of Chinese Art. c. 603)

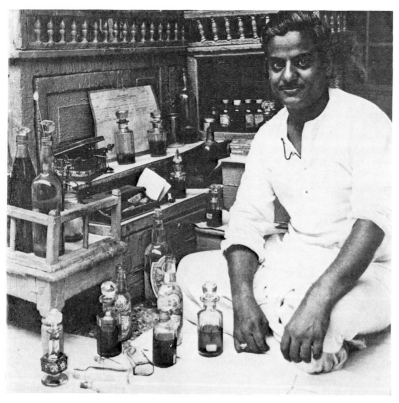

4. *MODERN INDIAN PERFUME SHOP*
Chandi Chowk, Delhi.

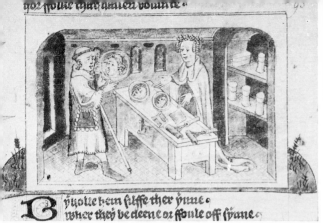

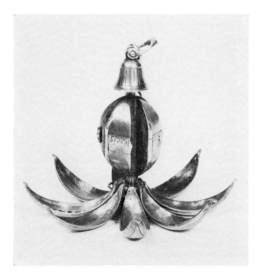

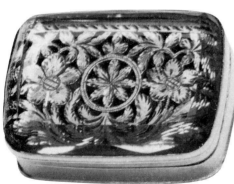

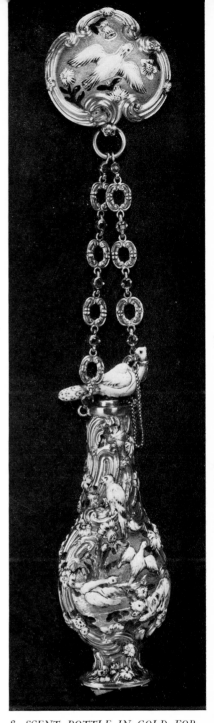

5. *(top) THE LADY HAGIOGRAPH DISPLAYING MIRRORS AND COSMETICS TO THE PILGRIM*
From G. de Duguiville's The Pilgrimage of the Life of Man, trans. by John Lydgate, 1426. (British Museum MS Cotton, Tiberius A VII)

6. *(middle) POMANDER, SILVER, 17TH CENTURY*
When closed it resembles an apple. Some segments are engraved with the names of spices. Height 7 cm. (Wellcome Institute of the History of Medicine)

7. *(below) VINAIGRETTE*
Silver, engraved with topaz cover, c. 1820. 4 × 3 cm.

8. *SCENT BOTTLE IN GOLD FOR ATTACHING TO BELT OR CHATE-LAINE, MID-18TH CENTURY*
Probably English though in Louis XV style, the bottle ornamented with a carnelian, flowers and doves, one of which surmounts the stopper: the gold chain embellished with precious stones and its gold head chased and decorated with flowers and a bird. (Leon Givaudan Collection. Photo: Raoul Foulon)

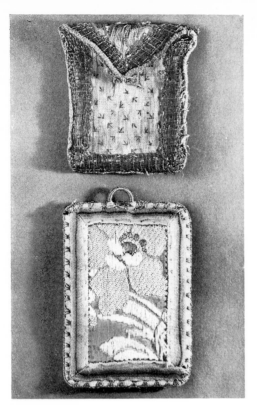

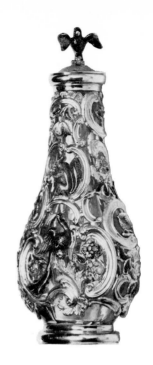

9. *(above, left)* PLAGUE SACHETS, CANTON OF LUCERNE, 17TH CENTURY
Made of embroidered silk, 9 × 7.5 and 7 × 5.5 cm. and containing medicinal herbs and printed plague charms. Schweitzerisches Pharmazie-historisches Museum, Basle. (From A History of Drugs *by Lydia Mez-Mangold)*

10. *(above, right)* SCENT BOTTLE, 19TH CENTURY
Cut glass, enamelled in rich colours. c. 1840. Height 13 cm.

11. *(below)* FRENCH PERFUMERS' COSMETIC JARS, 18TH CENTURY
All bear names of Paris perfumers. (The London Museum)

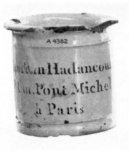

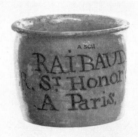

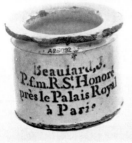

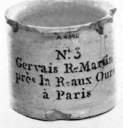

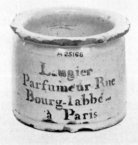

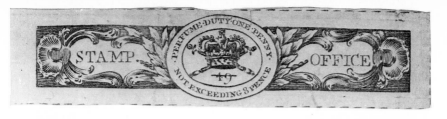

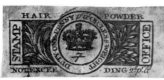
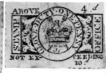

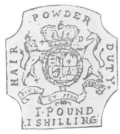

12. *(above)* BRITISH PERFUME AND HAIR POWDER STAMPS
Perfume Duty Stamp, 1786, One Penny (rare). Middle, left and right: Hair Powder Duty Stamps—
One Penny per pound on powder sold at under 2s. pound, 1796 (rare). Centre: Glove Duty Stamp—One
Penny on gloves priced between 4d and 10d., c. 1785. (Private Collection) Below: Guinea Stamp, embossed
in relief, on Annual Certificates to use Hair Powder. (From The Stamp Duty of Great Britain & Ireland,
a catalogue of embossed revenue stamps, 1694–1930, by S. B. Frank and Josef Schonfield)
13. *(below, left)* POMANDERS, SILVER, 17TH CENTURY
Vase shape with cover, engraved. Height 6 cm. Spinning top shape, diaper decoration. Height 10 cm. (Well-
come Institute of the History of Medicine)
14. *(below, right)* COTY PERFUME BOTTLE, c. 1910, Height 12 cm.
Designed by R. Lalique, Paris. (Coty Collection, London)

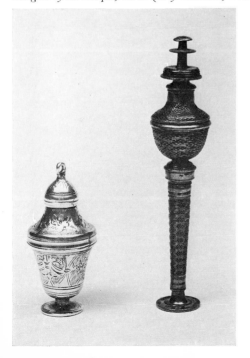

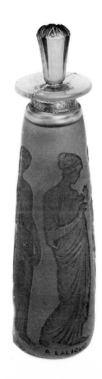

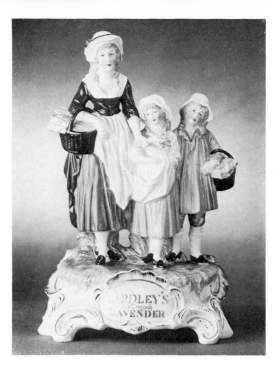

15. *YARDLEY LAVENDER SELLERS' GROUP,*
c. 1913
Originally designed as a Flower Seller's Group by Francis
Wheatley. Height 30 cm.

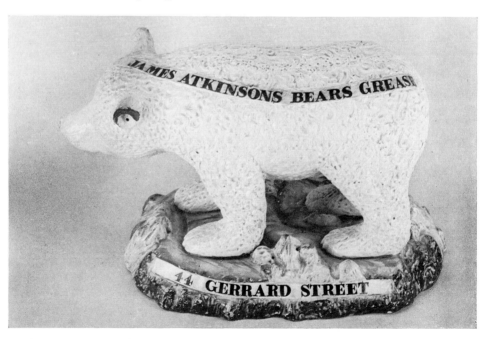

16. *JAMES ATKINSON'S BEAR, 19TH CENTURY*
White glazed earthenware, plinth coloured green and blue to imitate rocks and seaweed. Length 40 cm.
(Historical Collection: Pharmaceutical Society of Great Britain)

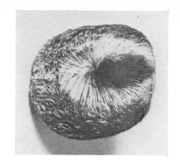

17. (right) MUSK POD
From the male musk deer.

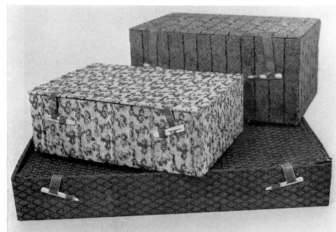

18. (left) MUSK CAD-
DIES, c. 1900–1910
Each holds one cati weight
approx. 1½ lb, of musk
pods, exported from China.
Boxes covered with cotton
embroidered in red designs,
one with print under lid
showing Chinese armed with
bows and arrows shooting
musk deer. All boxes fas-
tened with bone pins. Centre
box approx. 19.5 × 11.25
× 9 cm. (Private Collec-
tion)

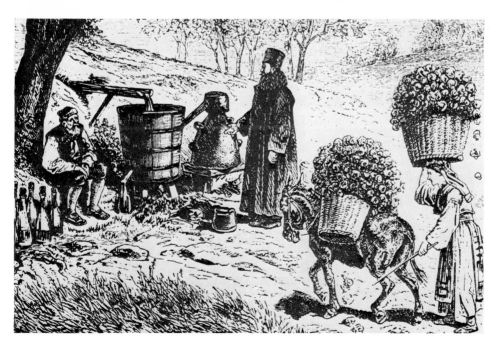

19. DISTILLATION OF ROSES IN KAZANLIK, BULGARIA, 19TH CENTURY
From woodcut by F. Kanitz. (Pharmachim State Economic Trust, Sofia, Bulgaria)

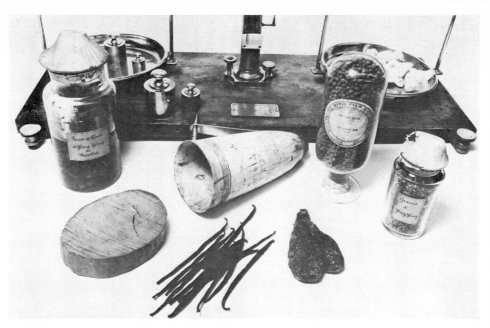

20. PERFUME MATERIALS
Back Row: Fruits and flowers of Ylang Ylang; Horn used for exporting Abyssinian civet; Piment noir from Jamaica; Truffles in the scale pan; Front Row: Sandalwood; Vanilla pods and Castor pods. (Guerlain Collection, Paris)

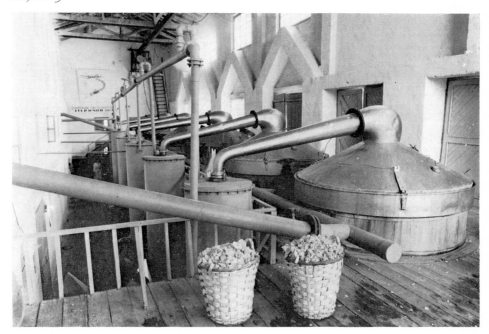

21. MODERN DISTILLATION EQUIPMENT FOR OTTO OF ROSE
(Pharmachim State Economic Trust, Sofia, Bulgaria)

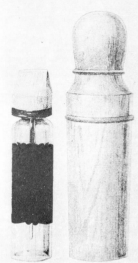

PHILIPPOPLE

(BULGARIE)

Tube bouchon émérie
avec tige, avec
étiquette de garantie
et etui bois:

No. 170 de 10 gr.
Frcs.   la pièce

Des flacons sans luxe sont
remplis par poids d'après le
désir de l'acheteur
          à Frcs.   le ko

Les prix sont au comptant et
franco de port si la commande
dépasse 100 Frcs.

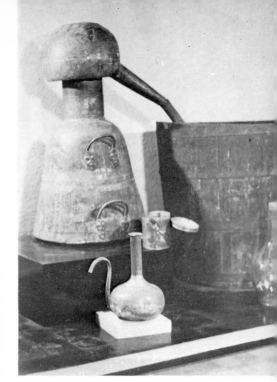

22. (above, left) SAMPLE BOTTLE OF OTTO OF ROSE, 20TH CENTURY
With its outer wooden container. Philippople, Bulgaria. (Pharmachim State Economic Trust, Sofia, Bulgaria)
23. (above, right) ALEMBIC FOR DISTILLATION USED IN BULGARIA, LATE 18TH CEN-
TURY
The illustration shows a wooden receiver with a laboratory flask. (Pharmachim State Economic Trust, Sofia,
Bulgaria)
24. (below) DRUM FOR THE EXPORT OF OTTO OF ROSE
These drums are known as 'konkouns'. On the left are modern glass flasks and containers for Otto samples.
(Pharmachim State Economic Trust, Sofia)

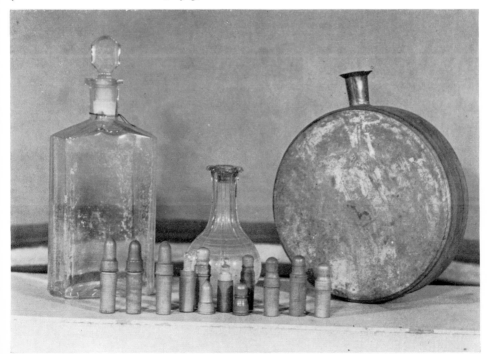

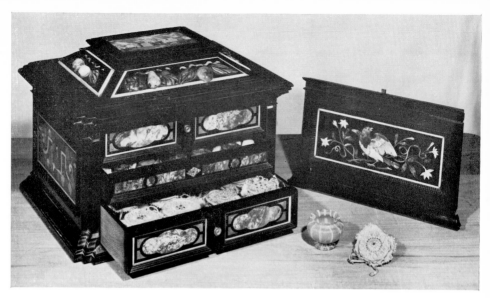

25. PERFUME CASE—FLORENTINE, 17TH CENTURY

Gift of the Grand Duke of Florence to Oliver, Lord Cromwell. This beautifully finished wooden casket, about 38 × 30.5 × 23 cm., decorated with variegated marble panels has a removable front panel revealing three drawers. The lower drawer is open to show eight Venetian glass pots, each with a fabric cover, in the centre of which semi-precious stones are sewn. (By courtesy of the Curator of the Cromwell Museum, Huntingdon. Photo: Edward Leigh, Cambridge)

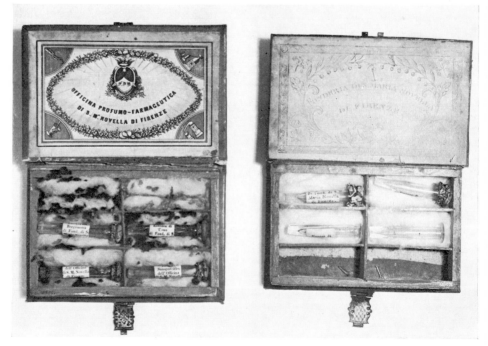

26. PERFUME CASES IN BOOK FORM CONTAINING FLORAL ESSENCES

Left: Officina Profumo-Farmaceutica di S. Maria di Firenze, 18th century, tooled leather cover. Right: Fonderia di S. Maria Novella di Firenze, 17th century, linen cover. (Wellcome Institute of the History of Medicine)

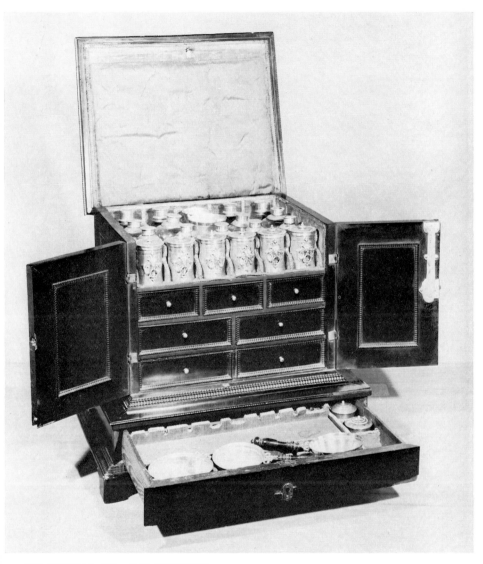

27. SURGEON'S CASE, 18TH CENTURY

Fitted with ornamental unguent pots, instruments and bleeding bowl. (Cromwell Museum, Huntingdon. Photo: Edward Leigh, Cambridge)

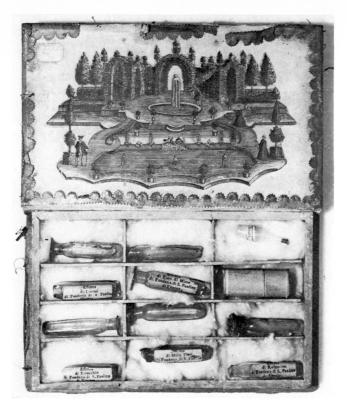

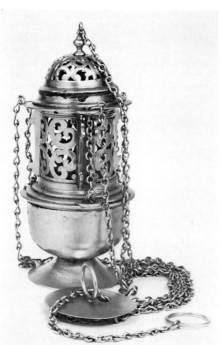

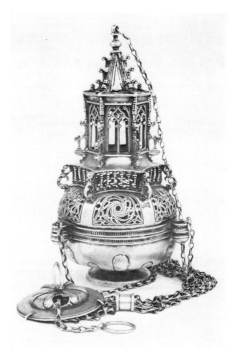

29. (left) SPANISH SILVER-GILT CENSER, c. 1600
Made in three parts. Engraved underneath in a modern hand 'From the chapel at Dilston Hall'.
Height 20 cm.
30. (right) PORTUGUESE SILVER CENSER, 16TH CENTURY
Gothic form. Height 24.5 cm.

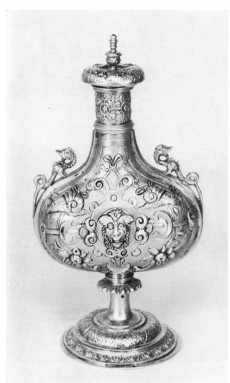

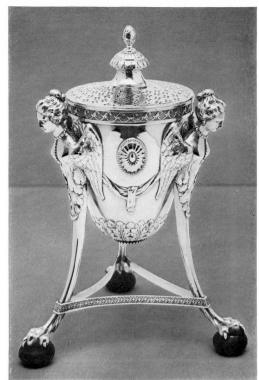

31. (above, left) ELIZABETHAN
SCENT FLAGON, LONDON, 1563
Height 17 cm. Weight 6 oz. 11 dwt.
32. (above, right) CASSOLETTE,
SILVER, 1779
Designed by Robert Adam and made by
Matthew Boulton, Height 20 cm. (From
The Great Silver Manufactory by Eric
Delieb)

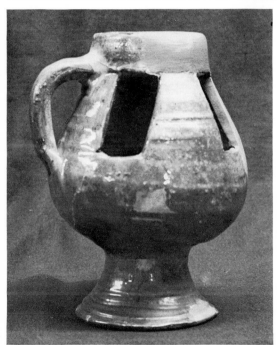

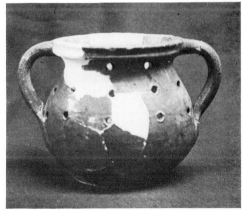

33. (left) FUMING POT, EARTHENWARE, LATE 16TH CENTURY
Light green glaze. One handle missing. Height 22 cm. Excavated in Southampton by F. A. Aberg. (God's
Tower Museum, Southampton)
34. (right) FUMING POT, EARTHENWARE, LATE 17TH OR EARLY 18TH CENTURY
Brown-green glaze. Height 12 cm. Excavated in Southampton by J. Wacher. (God's Tower Museum,
Southampton)

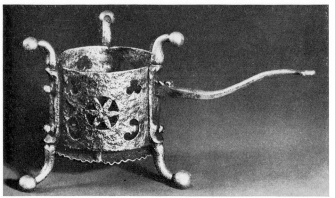

35. IRON FUMIGATOR,
18TH CENTURY
*Height 7 cm. Schweitzeri-
sches Pharmazie-historisches
Museum, Basle. (From* A
History of Drugs *by Lydia
Mez-Mangold)*

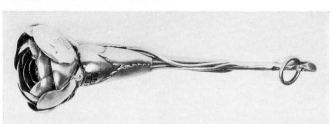

36. GOLD VINAI-
GRETTE IN THE FORM
OF A ROSE, 18TH CEN-
TURY
*Length 8 cm. (Wellcome
Institute of the History of
Medicine)*

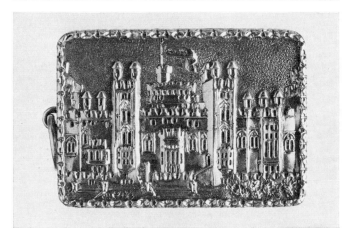

37. VINAIGRETTE,
SILVER, GEO. III
*Depicts Windsor Castle in
relief. 4 × 3 cm. (Well-
come Institute of the History
of Medicine)*

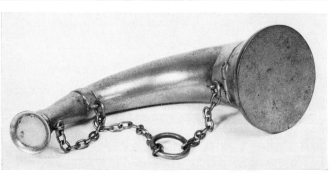

38. VINAIGRETTE,
SILVER HUNTING
HORN, c. 1860
*Made by S. Morden & Co.,
London. Length 10 cm.
(Wellcome Institute of the
History of Medicine)*

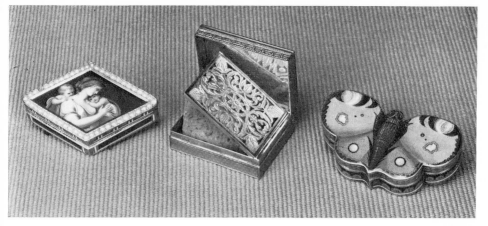

39. VINAIGRETTES, 18TH CENTURY
*(Left to right): Pearl framed, lozenge shape with enamelled
cover, French Directoire style. Gold, enamelled, with view of
Geneva on the cover. Butterfly form enamelled in natural colours
with base and side in blue, made in Geneva. (Leon Givaudan
Collection. Photo: Raoul Foulon, Paris)*

*40. (right) VINAIGRETTE, OPALINE GLASS, 19TH
CENTURY*
*Decorated in enamel, the fingers crossed over the thumb to avert
the Evil Eye. Height 10 cm. (Wellcome Institute of the History
of Medicine)*

*41. (below) SCENT BOTTLES IN GOLD AND ENAMEL,
18TH CENTURY*
*Left to right: Dresden pear shaped, decorated in Watteau style,
the stalk and leaf gilded, the upper part with naturalistic pine-
apple design. Battersea enamel, the base hexagonal, blue ground
with flowers in reserved panels and dove closure. Probably French,
baluster shaped bottle in gold, Regency style, chased and enamelled,
the panels with domestic animal scenes. Probably French, enamelled
in green and ornamented with flowers in gold and with porcelain
stopper, gold mounted. (Leon Givaudan Collection. Photo: Raoul
Foulon, Paris)*

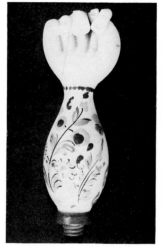

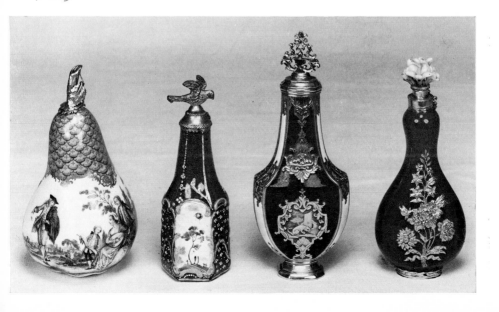

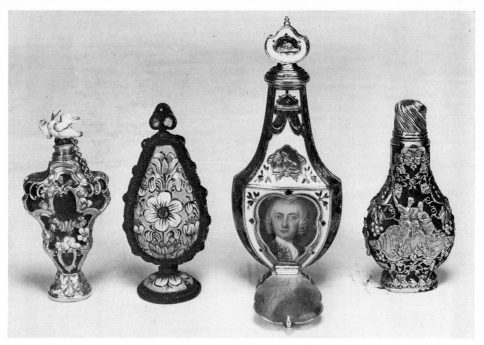

42. SCENT BOTTLES IN GOLD AND ENAMEL, 18TH CENTURY

Left to right: English, gold chased and enamelled. The base in carnelian provides a seal in the form of a man's hand. Bottle in the form of an olive, made of two enamelled plaques in blue on which flowers in white and yellow are enclosed in a setting of silver with garnets and rhinestones. Clover-leafed stopper similarly jewelled. French Regency, Gold bottle in baluster form, the upper part and the stopper decorated with the fox and grapes and other scenes. One side opens to reveal the head of a man. French, Louis XV period, gold bottle, chased and enamelled with Watteau figures on a cask and vine decoration. (Leon Givaudan Collection. Photo: Raoul Foulon, Paris)

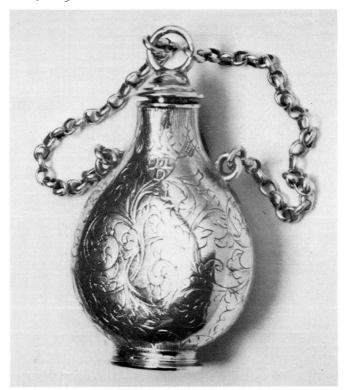

43. *(left)* SCENT BOT-
TLE, SILVER, WIL-
LIAM & MARY PERIOD
Engraved, with silver chain.

herbs. In the eighteenth century many Judges and officials connected with the law died after contracting jail fever because of contact with prisoners who had been in jail in insanitary conditions for some months before being tried. The Lord Chief Baron Pengelly was a victim at Taunton in 1730. At the Old Bailey, London, the Lord Mayor and others succumbed in 1750. This led to the custom of strewing herbs in the Courts and the carrying of nosegays.[6] In the *Life of Sir Edward Wild*, a former Recorder of the City of London, the author states that the posies or nosegays should contain seven herbs: balm, camomile, hyssop (caper), wild marjoram, rosemary, rue and sage, and additionally be scented with lavender, wallflowers and rose.[7]

In France during the seventeenth century there were many novelties. A new method of perfuming rooms started during the time of Anne of Austria (d. 1666), wife of Louis XIII and mother of Louis XIV, and who acted as Regent during her son's infancy. Up to her time the strewing of sweet-smelling herbs and barks was the usual means of perfuming rooms but she had small cages of artificial birds, made out of perfumed pastes, lozenge or bird shape, suspended from the ceilings. These were called 'Oiselets de Chypre', and were heavily scented. They could also be burnt in a chafing dish. Lemery[8] said they were called 'oiselets' because they rose up in the air when set alight, and 'Chypre' because Cyprus was the place where heavy perfumes originated and the lozenges were better made there than elsewhere. The craze for these oiselets was almost over by the end of the century.

It was about this period that scent sachets, small cushions filled with scented powders for use in the house or to be carried in the pocket (Sachets a la Roy) were being superseded by sachets filled with rose petals and other flowers and herbs. Sachets filled with medicinal herbs and printed charms had formerly been used as a protection against plague. The name pot pourri was given to these floral sachets. By the eighteenth century specially shaped vases were being made in gold, silver or porcelain, with pierced holes in the upper part and the lid so that when placed

---

[6] Tanner, E. S., *May It Please your Lordship*, London, 1971.

[7] Blackman, R. J., *Life of Sir Edward Wild*, London, 1935, 201–4.

[8] Lemery, Nicolas, *Pharmacopée Universelle*, Paris, 1690. The 5th ed., Paris, 1763, also contained formulae for these oiselets. Moise Charas, apothecary to Charles II, gives formulae for fumigating pastilles and oiselets in his *Pharmacopée Royale*, Paris, 1676. His alternative method of using them was to mix the powdered pastille with scented water and to pour this mixture on to a hot chafing dish.

in a room the perfume could diffuse. In the middle of the century the pot-pourri vase was so much in demand that the perfumers of France adopted it as their symbol, reproducing it upon their trade cards and handbills. Elegant ladies made up the contents of their own vases. The vases were often styled cassolettes though that name was more usually applied to the same type of vessel in which aromatic lozenges were ignited to fumigate rooms. Vessels of more robust design were made in iron.

In France during the seventeenth century nothing was too far-fetched for improving the complexion of the ladies of the Court—almonds, bread-crumbs, ceruse, sublimate or rouge of Spain. No wonder the toilette be-came a grand affair when every lady's dressing table was crammed with bottles and pots. A special '*bleu de veine*' was offered to those who wanted to emphasize the veins on their breasts. This was made of Briancon chalk coloured with Prussian blue. The use of a water to blanch the skin was followed by a lotion to give it a pink colour or if a dark skin was preferred that too could be managed with a dye. There was gold hair powder for the rich and for the less wealthy, one of powdered copper.

Even the young Louis XIV took a hand in preparing perfumes for his august person in the boutique of the famous Martial, the Court perfumer who wrote poems. This annoyed Molière who asked: 'Can he write too, I thought he was a perfumer'. Most of the Paris perfumers at that time had their boutiques near the Pont St Michel: it was only later they moved to the St Honoré quarter. Many named their preparations after important people such as the 'Eau de Ninon de l'Enclos', in honour of the celebrated beauty of the seventeenth century, noted for her Salon of distinguished men and women. The French Gantiers-Parfumeurs could find all the recipes needed for their pomades, essences and the perfuming of gloves from one of the Masters, Simon Barbe, whose *Le Parfumeur Royal*, Paris, 1699, had everything, including the preparation of the highly scented tobaccos then in fashion.

Once Louis XV (1710–1774) was really his own master and had control of his Court, Versailles became a byword for the use of perfume and it well deserved its name of Le Cour Parfumé. At Vincennes and Sèvres there were enormous fountains of perfumes mounted in gilt bronze and decorated with statues and bouquets of flowers. Even the wainscoting of rooms had to be perfumed. There was such competition for busi-ness amongst the Gantiers-Parfumeurs that orders were given that they should sell only what they themselves produced and only in their own boutiques.

Amongst the novelties was the introduction of soaps made in moulds and the fashioning of coffrets, called 'Necessaires porte-parfume', to hold two, three or four small bottles of perfume. Their invention is attributed to Galuchat who made them in sharkskin, green or grey. The English chose to call this roughened skin shagreen. With the glass phials, gold stoppered, was a tiny funnel for pouring from a larger vessel. Coffrets could be obtained in many shapes and with applied or repoussé decoration, in porcelain decorated with rural scenes or birds and flowers or enamelled. An alternative was to put the phials in a morocco leather case tooled to resemble a small book. Large sized coffrets to hold a dozen pots of rouge or creams were available and many were specially made for celebrities. Certainly Madame la Marquise de Pompadour, favourite of Louis XV, would have made use of all the beauty aids then offered by the Court perfumers.

The eighteenth century began a new period for the United Kingdom. After Queen Anne came the Hanoverians and with them the beginnings of industrialization, less dependance upon French fashions, more insistence upon home decoration for the wealthy and the middle classes, using furniture designed by Chippendale, Sheraton, and Robert Adam, the introduction of English porcelain, beautiful silverware—all combining to add to the appearance of elegance and good manners. Naturally this created additional interest in personal adornment. The tradesmen's cards of the century show the extent to which perfumers catered for all classes. They offered powders, perfumed waters, essences, oils, soaps, washballs, pomatums, pastes, powder bags and powdering machines, and a score of other preparations and articles designed chiefly for the ladies. Those who cultivated the wearing of a toupee could have French Roll Pomatum for it with fillets and black pins for the hair, and paper cauls to wear under wigs. If they were so minded, 'Cloud ditaliee' to burn in their rooms.

Mention has been made above of the practice of the Italians a century before of putting up tiny bottles of choice essences packed in the form of books. In 1777 bottles of perfumes made up into little books were still being advertised by Lewis and David Bourgeois of the Haymarket, London. Along with these the intending purchaser could make choice of a 'Variety of Cut-Glass, Ivory, Tortoiseshell, Dog-skin, and other Smelling bottles' in addition to cheese, Switzerland tea, and herbs for treating wounds. The Bourgeois brothers seem to have had a share in several businesses in or near the Haymarket. At first their trade sign was at the

Three Arquebusade Bottles which were depicted on their trade cards.*
Then came Bourgeois & Huguenin, with the same sign at No. 33 Haymarket: perfumers to their Royal Highnesses the Prince and Princess of
Wales and Prince William of Gloucester. About the same period Bourgeois,
Amick & Son, Perfumers to the Prince & Princess of Wales, and the Dukes
of Clarence and Sussex, at No. 32. A still further business was conducted
in the name of Bourgeois, Delacroix & Co. (formerly Bourgeois & Amick).

About this time D. Rigge, perfumer, who had been with a notable
master, Mr Richard Warren, whose pots and bottles come up for sale
now and again, but who now had his own perfumery warehouse in London,
was ready to supply the Nobility and Gentry with a Royal Compound
of violets and jessamin, to cause the hair to grow thick and strong, and
for those who needed it, a 'Hair Water for changing red or grey hair to
fine black or brown'.

The extent of the commerce in perfumes and cosmetics between
France and England during the second half of the eighteenth century is
well illustrated by the many white glazed earthenware pots bearing the
names of French perfumers, almost all established in Paris, which are to
be seen in museums here or which are found during archaeological ex-
cavations in towns. Although it has sometimes been assumed that these
pots, lettered with the names and addresses of French perfumers in black
or manganese, were usually those brought back by visitors to the French
capital, there is evidence of a large trade between Paris and London from
1750 to 1800.

In the eighteenth century the name of the French Guild or Corporation
of Perfumers was still that of Gantiers-Parfumeurs (Glovers-Perfumers),
formed in earlier times when the making and perfuming of gloves was
their main business. The names most often seen on the pots in England,(11)
which merit the attention of collectors, are:

Beauiard J. P.f.m. (perfumeur), R. St Honoré, près le Palais Royal à
Paris
Fargeon P.f.m. Rue de Roule à Paris
Chardin Hadancourt P.f.m. Pont Michel à Paris
Gervais R. Martin près la R.-Ours à Paris

---

* Arquebusade Water (Eau d'Arqubusade, Aqua Vulneria), in large square
shouldered bottles usually imported from Switzerland, was used for wounds, con-
tusions and ulcers. A complicated formula appeared in old Continental pharmacopoeias and continued at least until 1848. The arquebus was an early type of
portable gun supported upon a tripod or forked rest.

Lugier Parfumeur Rue Bourg-l'Abbé—à Paris

RAIBAUD R. St Honoré A Paris

Some of these names appear in the list of Merchant-Glovers, Powder Makers and Perfumers of the City, Faubourgs and Suburbs of Paris (Liste du Corps des Marchands-Gantiers-Poudriers-Parfumeurs de la Ville, Faubourgs et Banlieux de Paris) published for the year 1776.[9]

Jean-Joseph Gervais, rue St Martin, had been admitted to the Guild in 1745: he became a Jurist in 1758 and a Syndic in 1759. His son, Denis Barthelemi, was described as one of the 'Messieurs les Modernes', and had been elected a Master-perfumer in 1764.

Gabriel Leger Hadancourt, probably a son of Chardin Hadancourt, had been elected one of the Young Master-perfumers in 1767. Jean L. Fargeon, son of the more noted J. H. Fargeon, had his preliminary election to the Guild in 1774.

The J. H. Fargeon, Gantier-Parfumeur du Roi, whose shop was in the rue de Roule, Paris, and whose name appears on many pots, was a perfumer with a very large business comprising many kinds of pomades, perfumes, toilet waters, and assorted cosmetics. Alas, he was forced into bankruptcy in 1778, largely because he failed to get in the debts due to him.[10] These included the immense sum of £20,909 for perfumes and cosmetics supplied to the King, Louis XV, up to the date of his death in 1774, and whose debts to Fargeon had presumably accumulated and had not been paid by his successor, Louis XVI. Besides the debts due from the King there were recorded supplies to duchesses, chevaliers, countesses and others, most of whom would have been connected with the extravagances of Louis XV's Court.

Fargeon had a widespread business, supplying all kinds of goods to various cities in France and he sent dozens of the pots of the kind illustrated, to Mr Nicolle (or Nicole) of London, the invoices to whom totalled £16,455, and to a Mr Caty (£10,682) and to other London importers of French perfumery to a value of £5,778. The detailed list comprises 12 kinds of pomades, including pomade divine, frangipani, powder and pomade à Maréchale, essences, embroidered jasmin sachets and liquide à la Duchesse. There were lots of 1,000 pots of pomade invoiced at a time. The total indebtedness of the London importers amounted to £33,626 of which some £20,800 was recovered. Fargeon's debts amounted to almost a quarter

---

[9] Paris: Valleyre. n.d. Bibliothèque Historique de la Ville de Paris, No. 30325.

[10] Archives de la Seine, Paris, MS 2335–3–R. Faillite—Fargeon, J. H.

of a million pounds. He hoped to collect most of this sum but since his statement of accounts showed that the whole of his manufacturing equipment and raw materials in the factory had to be valued, it is questionable whether his creditors received all that was due to them. Nevertheless, his son became a Master-perfumer and doubtless retrieved something from a business conducted on such a wholesale scale. The original documents signed by J. H. Fargeon in a shaky hand suggest either increasing age or a nervous state induced by the bankruptcy.

Vinaigrettes

In 1720 Sir Richard Mead, a distinguished physician in England, practising during the first half of the seventeenth century, was asked to set out his views on combatting the plague. The scares were not yet over and there was fear of its return. Mead condemned the use of the aromatics that had made up the pomanders and instead strongly urged the adoption of wine and vinegars as better preventives.[11] Already in France rue or other herbs had been steeped in vinegar[12] for the use of which specially made containers were on sale. His recommendations, coming from one of the leading men in the country, was heeded. Pomanders went out and vinaigrettes, so-called because of the French name, came in. The idea was quickly adopted, vinaigrettes became the fashionable things to have as objets d'art, if for no other reason, and jewellers made them in gold, silver-gilt, silver, sometimes covered with a semi-precious stone such as topaz or other translucent material to set off the cover below.(7) Shapes and designs varied enormously. As long as the principal object was achieved, the cases could be of any kind that caught the fancy of the owner. Thus we find them made as shells, watches, books, handbags, or more com-

---

[11] Mead, Richard, *A Short discourse concerning pestilential contagion and the methods used to prevent it*, London: S. Buckly, 1720.

[12] A prophylactic vinegar, known as 'Marseilles' or 'Four Thieves' Vinegar', was prepared by steeping various herbs, lavender flowers, garlic, cinnamon, cloves and nutmeg in strong vinegar for twelve days. After straining, a small quantity of camphor dissolved in spirits was added to the liquid. Modifications of this formula appeared in the *Edinburgh Pharmacopoeia* of 1817 and in the *Prussian Pharmacopoeia* of 1847. (In the mid-nineteenth century, Eugène Rimmel, a French perfumer established in London, developed the 'Thieves Vinegar' and presented it as a Toilet Vinegar. It was a best seller for many years, and is again on the market.)

monly, as thin rectangular boxes, about 4 × 2.5 cm., for carrying in the pocket or in purse or bag, and decorated by chasing, engraving or turning. Small chains were attached to many vinaigrettes for convenience and perhaps to avoid loss.

Not all vinaigrettes were made of costly metals: cheaper varieties could be obtained. All had a tightly-fitting cover: those of hard stones had metal mounts—an inner hinged grid, fretted or pierced, to prevent the escape of the piece of Turkey sponge soaked in aromatic vinegar and to allow the contents to be sniffed. The interior and the inner grid were usually gilt to prevent the action of the vinegar on the metal. Some of the vinaigrettes offered for sale will be seen to have retained portions of the original sponge.

Hair Powder

There was a need for hair powder for about 200 years, either for cleaning the wig, cleansing the head when the wig was off or in the Georgian era, when powdered wigs were in fashion, to produce a grey-white appearance. The long curled wigs of the time of Charles II and William III were worn in their natural colours. Charles seems to have copied his style from Louis XIV. Simpler styles were needed when hunting and for a period, the bag wig was the mode.

The nobility had their powder specially perfumed to their choice. The royal apothecary who supplied King William III was careful to write in his daybook whether he had sent the specially perfumed kind, at 20d per pound or the ordinary at 16d. For William too, he supplied a particular hand washing powder made of starch and oil of green almonds.

Throughout the eighteenth century perfumers advertised a variety of hair powders, scented with musk, rose and the like or non-scented. These could be obtained in different colours, white or grey being the most favoured. Gold dust was often used by ladies. For those whose hair was powdered by their maids or by valets, powdering masks were in use to prevent complexions or clothes being covered with powder by a too energetic servant.

Hair powder was subjected to tax in 1786. A duty upon all toilet preparations was imposed of 1½d on packages up to 1s face value, 1s on 5s and over. This duty was paid by the affixing of stamps to the package.(12) The dutiable list of some 200 items included 'Sweet Scents,

Odours, Perfumes, Cosmetics and Dentifrices'. Common soap was exempt. Hair powder, cold cream, wash balls, bear's grease and a few others could be stocked without affixing duty stamps until they were sold. The sellers had to take out an annual licence costing 1s and were obliged to have the words 'Licensed to deal in Perfumery' displayed on the front of their shops. It was soon apparent that the cost of collecting the tax was too high when compared with the revenue it brought in. The tax was therefore repealed in 1800 but many preparations remained taxable and in 1802 a new Act listed, amongst other items, lip salves, dentifrices and particularly mentioned Hemet's Essence of Pearl Dentrifrice.

Though the tax on hair powder and cosmetics generally was repealed, there was still in existence another tax that Pitt had introduced to bring in funds to the Treasury. The Act of 1795, enforced from 5 May, imposed an obligation upon every person who used any kind of hair powder to take out a certificate or licence and pay a fee of one guinea for it.(12) The list of persons holding licenses had to be posted on church doors. License holders quickly became known as 'guinea pigs'. Householders had to make out a list of persons in their dwelling houses who used hair powder and surveyors were appointed to inspect houses for the purpose of reporting offenders. There was a special rate for the householder who paid the tax for two daughters: no tax was payable in respect of further daughters. Naturally the Royal House, their servants, and the Forces were exempt. The Act remained in force until 1869 though in 1801 the duty payable was assessed by the Commissioners of Taxes and certificates were discontinued.

The imposition of this tax came as a gift to the caricaturists of the day. Gillray, for example, had on sale even a month before the tax was imposed, a cartoon 'Leaving off Powder or the Frugal Family saving the guinea'. This showed a family of four, a father in old-fashioned dress with a small unpowdered wig sadly reading about the new tax in the *Gazette*; mother aghast as being offered an unpowdered wig; cropped-headed son and copper-haired daughter with no powder to cover the red tint. Isaac Cruickshank and others made much play with the 'guinea pigs', tilting at Pitt and Fox with caustic lampoons. By 1800 there were few left, men or women, who did not prefer their own hair to wigs and who did not follow the new classic style made fashionable by Napoleon's campaigns in Italy and Egypt.

4

Nineteenth Century to Modern Times

NAPOLEON'S assumption of the title of Emperor of France in 1804 and the creation of the First Empire which lasted until 1815, saw the resumption of Court life that had been in abeyance during the Revolution. The luxury trades could flourish again. The Empress Josephine, having been born in Martinique, never lost her inclination for the heavy scents associated with that Island. The ladies of the Court followed her example in having complexions heightened greatly by colour. Napoleon disliked a pale face—looking like a corpse was his rebuke—and large bills for rouge were submitted by perfumers such as Madame Martin whose establishment became known as 'le Rouge de la Cour' and Veuve Fargeon et Fils. Madame Fargeon was the widow of the Fargeon whose name appears on many of the French cosmetic jars and whose bankruptcy has been noted in the previous chapter. Others who received royal patronage in this period were Lubin at the sign of Aux armes de France and whose rouge 'Sarkis' was regarded as the best for evening wear, and Houbigant, formerly Court perfumer to Louis XVI. It was Houbigant who devised the Parfum Recamier for the beautiful Madame Recamier who held sway until her death in 1849. Fads and fancies played a part in the cosmetic world and a Madame Tallier is credited with recommending the virtues of baths of strawberries and raspberries for improving the skin. Napoleon himself was a fervent believer in friction with Eau de Cologne and insisted upon being brushed down with it from head to foot, using 60 bottles a month. Even if he cared little for the occupants of Windsor Castle he consistently used Windsor soap.

During the romantic period in France which began in the first quarter of the century new preparations were introduced and Madame Lebrun established the first Institut de Beauté as a salon in the Place Vendôme, Paris. So successful was this that many more were started in France and they were copied in South America.

It was a period when rapid technical improvements in production were initiated. By the middle of the century large-scale manufacture was advancing using newly invented machinery. What had formerly been small businesses grew into an industry. All through the century France led the way and kept her strong lead over competitors in other countries. The catalogues of perfume houses now offered a wide selection of all kinds.

Many of the numerous French perfumers of the nineteenth century have gained world-wide reputation. The eighteenth century had seen the establishment of Revillon in 1734, Houbigant in 1775 and Lubin in 1798. Revillon began as furriers in 1732 but soon entered the perfume industry. Pierre Francois Lubin (1774–1853), whilst still a pupil perfumer invented and sold his Eau de Lubin, the toilet water which was the foundation of a prosperous business. Jean-Francois Houbigant is said to have begun his career in Paris by carrying a basket of flowers. Hence his sign 'a La Corbeille des Fleurs' at No. 19 Faubourg St Honoré, where he was both perfumer and glove maker as was then customary. By 1801 he styled himself 'Marchand Parfumeur' though he still sold gloves. In the heyday of the *Muscadins*, just after the Revolution, so-named because they were so heavily perfumed with musk, their necks buried in high stocks, Houbigant flourished as never before. In 1829 his son, Armand-Gustave, was appointed perfumer to HRH Princess Adélaide d'Orléans, with the right to exhibit her coat of arms over his shop. This and his patronage by the Empress Eugènie in 1860, put Houbigant amongst the leading Paris Perfumers. Early in the nineteenth century came Ed. Pinaud and Laugier Père et Fils and not long after were Gellé Frères, 1826, Guerlain 1828, Bourgeois 1840, Molinard 1849, L. T. Piver by 1850, Worth* in 1858, Roger & Gallet, successors to J. M. Farina in 1862, and at the end of the century or a little later, Francois Coty, Chanel, Vigny, Lanvin and a host of others. Laugier Père, having succeeded to the business of Fargeon Jeune in 1826 brought out a Savon Egyptian especially for the military to promote the growth of moustaches. When André Bourgeois first made his Poudre de Riz de Java at his house in Paris in 1840 and trundled a barrow through the streets selling it, he hoped only to make a living: never for a moment did he think he had the capacity to found a business that would lead to international trade. For more than eighty years his

---

* It was John Philip Worth, son of an Englishman and a successful dressmaker to the Empress Eugénie, who had the idea that perfumes and the Haute Couture organized by his brother would go well together. This was the beginning of an international business.

Poudre de Riz remained the leading face powder, so well established that for a century the type of box and the labels were unchanged.

The fine perfume makers of the late nineteenth century realized the need for the special packaging of choice perfumes. The appeal to the eye of shapes of bottles, ribbons, delicately placed labels, the whole in a coffret lined with silk or velvet, the interior moulded to the bottle, all added to the attractiveness of the perfume itself. The principal glass houses making scent bottles in a host of varied designs have been Cristalleries de Baccarat, (established in Lorraine in 1764), Cristalleries de Nancy, Cristalleries de Saint-Louis, (formed in 1767 and in 1781 the first to begin manufacture of sparkling crystal), André Jolivet, Verreries d'Argenteuil, and Viard et Viollet le Duc. Most of these also furnished the glass services de toilette when those were in fashion. The real presentation de luxe came with M. Francois Coty in 1905. His demands on the Cristalleries de Baccarat revolutionized the ideas of the perfume industry in their search for new designs. He is said to be not only the promoter of the revolution but actually its dictator. It was Coty who in 1910 invited René Lalique, one of the great masters in Art Nouveau, to create new forms. These included tall mushroom-stoppered bottles of square section, round bottles decorated with studding in the form of limpets picked out in contrasting colours, and half-round bottles of orange segment shape decorated with rows of contrasting mulberry-shaped blobs. Engraved bottles of mushroom or sea-urchin shape were made for Worth. Some of these early pieces bear the signature 'R. Lalique, France', as was customary on the Lalique art glass.(14)

Other French designers of scent bottles at this period were the decorators Sue et Mare—a black octagonal bottle with spherical stopper is typical of their work, and Maurice Martinot, whose outstanding designs were personal and therefore restricted in quantity and whose pieces were signed. Throughout the whole of the Art Nouveau period the manufacturer, influenced by the current mode, constantly tried to give the purchaser the kind of bottle and pack that was in keeping with the prevalent artistic ideas.

The French revival of luxuries after the Revolution had its repercussions in Britain. Well before the end of the eighteenth century there were many describing themselves as perfumers within the boundaries of the City of London and in the developing Bond Street area. Some of these combined the sale of perfumery with other profitable merchandise. Mr William Tremlett's sister, who succeeded her brother, sold 'all sorts of snuff and perfumes' at the Young Civet Cat near the Temple. James D. Smyth, whose sign was also the Civet Cat, of New Bond Street, took his nephews into the business: they became perfumers to George III.*(85) That monarch, judging by the claims made on tradesmen's billheads, must have appointed several perfumers. Hairdressing was often combined with the selling of perfumery. Stewart of Old Broad Street, a perfumer to the King and to the Prince of Wales, advertised his book on the 'Whole Art of Hairdressing'. Packwood, in the City of London, dressed ladies' hair elegantly for one shilling, powder and pomade included. Dighton, who had been sworn perfumer to George I, was to be found at the corner of Fleet Street. Perfumers bearing foreign names who flourished at this time included P. Grellier who added to perfumery the importation of Alderney cows for His Royal Highness the Prince of Wales; August Loriot, perfumer, was also a stationer and toy man; and Sanguine, well known for his bear's grease and who besides hardware sold decorated pocket books. Mrs Hare l'Aigle, successor to Madme de Bresson, sold 'The True and Genuine Rouge'.

The outburst of perfumers amongst the luxury trades expanded during the nineteenth century, helped no doubt by the extravagances of the well-to-do under the leadership of the Prince of Wales, later George IV. Andrew Pears, a Barber-Surgeon, started the business which became A. and F. Pears, in 1789. He modestly advertised in *Bell's Weekly Messenger* in 1810 that 'by a curious chemical process' his Soap was purified from all noxious substances. In 1799 a young man named James Atkinson set out to walk from Cumberland to London to make a fortune. His entrance into the atmosphere of perfumery has all the air of romance. As his sole companion he travelled with a bear: the selling of perfumed bear's grease as a hair pomade was his proposed means of livelihood.

Atkinson, established at 44 Gerrard Street, London, is said to have chained his bear outside to attract custom. Whether true or not, he prospered, selling pots of grease with lids picturing a bear. Before he left Soho for New Bond Street he had models of a bear made in white pottery: these he may have distributed to retailers who stocked his product.(16) He launched out into hair dyes, soaps and perfumes and in 1826 became one of the perfumers to the Royal Family. To suit the mode he made pastilles for burning in his 'Philosophical Incense Burner', and he began

* Robert Butcher, the Duke of Bedford's chief agent, has left a record of purchases in 1757 from James Smyth & Co. of perfumed soap, powder, pomade and lavender water. (*The Russells in Bloomsbury* by Gladys Scott Thomson, London, 1940, 277-9.)

to make his own brands of Lavender Water and Eau de Cologne. Joined by his brother Edward in 1831, hence the name J. & E. Atkinson, by 1832 the partnership became firmly established in Old Bond Street at the corner of Burlington Gardens. Here a palatial display attracted the fashionable world. Here too, until World War II, from the belfry of the new Atkinson Building could be heard the famous carillon. Both brothers had died in the middle of the nineteenth century and were succeeded by a new generation of Atkinsons. Export trade began and manufacture was set up overseas. In 1941 the businesses of Atkinson and Erasmic were amalgamated. Atkinsons celebrated their 150th anniversary in 1949.

In 1970 the House of Yardley celebrated its 200th anniversary. It was in 1801 that William Yardley's daughter, Hermina, married William Cleaver, heir to an important soap and perfumery business dating from 1770. Yardley, himself a sword cutler, was guarantor for his son-in-law and took over that business which included the supply of lavender besides cosmetics and soap. The 'Yardley' Lavender Water became so important that in 1913 the Francis Wheatley Flower group, one of his set of 13 'Cries of London', was adapted for the widely distributed Old English Lavender Model and was then adopted as a trade mark for all the firm's lavender products.(15)

John Gosnell & Co., 1834, had an ancestry back to 1769 at least, when John Price first described himself as a perfumer. By 1832 Price and Gosnell became perfumers to the Royal family. New perfumery manufacturers were establishing themselves. At the beginning of this century firms like Grossmith & Co. had come into prominence with an 'Eastern' series such as 'Phul Nana' and 'Shem-el-Nessim'.

Once Leblanc had invented his process for making soda, manufacturers could produce soap on a large scale, discarding the old methods using wood-ash or ashes from burnt seaweed. Toilet soaps in varying degrees of quality were now available, finely milled, coloured, and perfumed to suit the user and in luxury packs as his purse permitted.

The Great Exhibition held in London in 1851 illustrated in no uncertain way the forward leaps which industrialization had taken during the first half of the nineteenth century and which continued unabated thereafter. It was in that year that William Bush set out to provide other manufacturers with distilled essences of natural products. By 1890 the firm of W. J. Bush & Co. were beginning to set up factories abroad, in Sicily, in Melbourne, Moscow and Grasse. Other British firms who were or who came into the field included Stafford Allen & Sons and Boake Roberts &

Co. These and others added synthetic compounds to their ranges of essences from cultivated plants and herbs so as to provide the perfumery, food and tobacco industries with most of the materials needed, including all kinds of artificial flavourings.

During the nineteenth century some perfumers who had started in France found Britain such a good market that they decided to make London their principal base. Of these, Septimus Piesse was both perfumer and technical writer. In one of his books he gives the formula for 'Bouquet of Buckingham Palace'. Eugène Rimmel, a Frenchman born in Paris in 1820 and son of a perfumer trained by Lubin, came to London to join his father in 1834, succeeding to the business in 1842. Rimmel's Fountain of Perfumery at the Great Exhibition put him in the front rank. From that time he issued annually calender-sachets in colour; now greatly prized. His *History of Perfumes* issued in 1865 was a best seller. He mentions the then new system of perfuming theatres: this was to pass steam through a concentrated essence and allow it to spread through the atmosphere. Rimmel was proud of the fact that his first premises were in Beaufort Building in the Strand, the address which in the first half of the eighteenth century had been that of the most notable London Perfumer of the time, Charles Lillie, whose trade bill bore a print of the Civet Cat and the City of Barcelona. Lillie's range of perfumes, soaps and cosmetics was extensive. He was a contributor to the *Spectator* and he gathered notes on his professional work which illness prevented him from publishing. The notes, edited by C. Mackenzie, finally appeared in 1822 as *Lillie's British Perfumer*. His editor says that Lillie in his day was the only man residing in London who had been regularly initiated and bred to the business of perfumery. Lillie's notes are comprehensive and mention explosive pastilles, filled with gunpowder, and suitable as a Christmas diversion. In his view the best face powder was made by grinding pearls to a fine powder. He tells how to make and perfume chicken skin gloves, extremely thin and costly.

Novels and plays of the eighteenth century made much of the 'vapours' to which ladies were prone. A useful antidote to this distressing condition, sometimes merely assumed, was the application to the nose of smelling salts. Originally prepared by distilling harts' horn shavings, which resulted in a strong ammonia, scented oils were added to cover the ammonia fumes and provide a more attractive preparation. An alternative was to mix ammonium carbonate with chalk and to dissolve this in water. Small pellets of sal prunella (fused potassium nitrate) might be added to the bottles. Throughout the nineteenth century and especially during the second half, smelling-salts bottles could be had in a variety of sizes, for handbag, made in white or coloured glass, often engraved. These were the rule until double-ended bottles, with gold, gilt or silver caps, also in a variety of colours became an accepted style. The cut outer casing of glass of one colour revealed the white or alternative colour beneath. These were common in the 1850s, and as antiques, are now eagerly collected. Hall marks on the silver caps readily serve to date them.

By 1880 even the country chemists in Britain, the chief sellers of perfumes and cosmetics up to that time, were advertising new proprietary perfumes in almanacks and were offering aromatic ozonizers, pine and eucalyptus air purifiers and perfumed calendars.

The change in hair fashion in the styles of wigs of the eighteenth century led to elaborate hairdressing in the 1770s. This gave an opening to the pomade makers. The dandies of the day, especially those who cultivated the macaronic styles of swept-up or swept-down hair needed pomades and oils. Whilst the caricaturists were making them a laughing stock, shrewed business men saw their opportunity. A. Rowland & Son of Hatton Garden, London, for example, made a fortune from the sale of their Macassar Oil, introduced about 1800 and described as 'The Original and Genuine', to ornament and embellish the human hair. According to the *Constitutional* for 1817, this consisted of olive or almond oil, coloured red with alkanet root, to which perfumed oils were added. By the 1850s Rowlands were reputed to be spending up to £20,000 a year on advertising, an unheard-of sum for those days.

Toilet Waters

Many of the Toilet Waters in general use during the nineteenth century were prepared either by distilling the water in which flowers such as roses had been immersed for some days or by direct distillation, i.e. passing steam through the flowers suspended on trays and collecting the oil as a distillate. Alcohol and water were then added to the oil to make the finished preparation.

From the sixteenth century onwards distillation of the water in which fresh flowers or herbs had been soaked was the usual method of preparing scented waters.

The Queen of Hungary's Water, attributed on doubtful grounds to a recipe said to be in the writing of Queen Elizabeth of Hungary dated 1235, attained world wide use. This preparation, virtually a spirit of rosemary, was made by distilling fresh rosemary in alcohol. This was very popular during the eighteenth century. A Hungary Water warehouse, at the Black Boy & Comb in Fleet Street advertising fresh Hungary Water in large half-pint bottles at 1s. 3d in 1721, drew attention to the test for a genuine article: 'One spoonful turns a glass of water as white as milk, counterfeits only turn it a sky colour'. It was the rosemary oil in the preparation that caused the opalescence when added to water. Besides counterfeits, there were a number of competing preparations on the market, notably the French Eau de Luce, advertised in 1754 as imported from Paris and sold as a Volatile Essence for carrying in the pocket as a smelling bottle, 'stronger than many kinds of Salts, more fragrant than Lavender, Hungary or any other odoriferous water'.

The Toilet Waters having the greatest popularity during the nineteenth century were Eau de Cologne, Lavender Water, Florida Water (in the USA), Honey Water and Eau de Portugal.

1. EAU DE COLOGNE

When first sold, about the beginning of the eighteenth century, it bore the title Aqua Admirabilis (L'Eau Admirable), and only after some years did it acquire its French name of Eau de Cologne. Claims have been made by various members of the Farina family, of Italian origin, that their predecessors invented and owned the original formula—either Johann Maria Farina whose address was 'Opposite Julich's Platz, Cologne' or Jean-Paul Féminis who migrated to Cologne from Milan. From 1902 to 1907 legal clarification of the competing claims was sought; finally, in 1907 the Supreme Court of the German Empire found that Jean-Paul Féminis was the original inventor. Nevertheless, documents not before the Court were said to establish that it was J. M. Farina ('Opposite Julich's Platz') who was entitled to the honour.[1] In 1818 Jean-Marie Farina, a descendant of Féminis, proclaimed his rights by a series of coloured posters. His for-

---

[1] Irissou, L., 'Sur l'Origine de l'Eau de Cologne', *Rev. d'Hist. de la Pharm.* Paris, 1952, 262; also discussed by P. Le Mery, *ibid.*, 1952, 318. For an interview with a descendant of the original J. M. Farina 'Opposite Julich's Platz', see *The Chemist and Druggist,* London, 1875, *17*, 172–6.

mula was sold to a Mons. J. Collas from whom in 1862 the perfumery firm of Roger & Gallet of Paris acquired it.

Many perfumers have had great success in marketing their own brands of Eau de Cologne. Why it came so quickly into fashion and why it has retained its place is something of a mystery. The occupation of the Rhineland by France during the seven years' war, about 1760, is thought to have widened its popularity and to have stimulated other perfumers than those of Cologne to manufacture their own brands. The fragrance for which it is esteemed in large part comes from the oils of bergamot, lemon, orange flower and lavender or rosemary which, with rectified spirit, are usually regarded as the basic constituents of any Eau de Cologne.[2]

2. LAVENDER WATER

No other Toilet Water of England has achieved such a well-deserved reputation. Though called 'Lavender Water' it would be more correctly called 'Spirit of Lavender' since it is essentially a solution of lavender oil in alcohol but each perfumer makes his own modifications to the basic ingredients by adding other essential oils or essences to improve the perfume. In the seventeenth century and for long after, a spirit of lavender (or lavender 'water') was prepared by distilling the freshly-picked lavender heads which had been immersed for a few days in alcohol. To obtain the oil, the flowering heads are now steam distilled; the oil floats on the surface of the water which is syphoned off from below. Many perfumers prefer to use an oil which has been matured for up to three years.

3. HONEY WATER

This was a sweet scented spirit containing lemon peel, nutmegs, cloves, orange flowers and other aromatic ingredients. All these were distilled and musk, honey and other essences added, with saffron to produce a rich colour. The preparation, almost as well known in France as in England, was used both as a face lotion and as a medicine.

---

[2] Poucher, W. A., *Perfumes, Cosmetics & Soaps*, London, 1941, II, 299-300.

4. FLORIDA WATER

This, a great favourite in the USA, came to be used there almost as universally as Lavender Water in the British Isles. It is still considered by many to combine the fragrance of Lavender Water with that of Eau de Cologne.[3]

5. EAU DE PORTUGAL

This was a variant of Eau de Cologne, made by omitting the orange flower oil.

---

[3] About 1880 the New York Perfumery Co. of Florida and New York was promoting its Florida Water, describing it as 'Distilled from the Choicest Exotics', with a label in colour showing a fountain of perfume and flowers. A popular brand was that of Murray & Lanman, New York (formerly Lanman and Kemp).(65) During the Spanish–American War, 1899–1901, packages of this and similar preparations had to carry a US tax stamp.(81).

Processes and Materials Used

Preparation

EVEN the simplest perfume, for example, Lavender Water, has three or four additives to render it stable and pleasant to use. For the more sophisticated perfumes the number of ingredients needed to modify the basic constituents can be a dozen or more and they must be 'fixed' to ensure that the perfume will last and be as fragrant at the end as at the beginning. The art of making perfumes calls for a keen 'nose' on the part of the perfumer, and, if he is to create a new perfume, one with what is termed a new 'note', which every perfumer tries to invent, the range of additives, modifiers and fixatives may easily be increased to as many as fifty or sixty, once he has decided upon the basic oils, concretes or absolutes he intends to use as his starters. There is no lack of synthetics for him to employ; possibly the range is so wide that it itself hampers him in his search for something new which will be attractive. His host of bottles containing oils, essences, synthetics and fixatives, formerly arranged on shelves round him like the console of an organ, is in Britain now usually grouped in ranks in front of him but still referred to as the perfumer's 'organ'. The console placing of bottles is retained by many of the perfumers in Grasse.

Odour Classification

Many attempts to aid the perfumer by classifying types of odours have been made, both by practising perfumers and others. One of them, Septimus Piesse, of France, arranged all the natural perfumes in a rising musical scale of values. Another, Eugène Rimmel, based his on the empirical likeness of the pleasant flower odours, divided into 18 classes; this was extended by Cerbelaud. None of the attempts so far have been of much assistance in the search for new and distinctive perfumes.

Fixatives

Theophrastus of Eresos, a pupil of Aristotle, wrote in the third century AD: 'The composition and preparation of perfumes aim entirely at making odours last'. To achieve this lasting fragrance the perfumer must know what will 'hold' the scent that will come from his blend of materials and what will increase its intensity. Here he has a choice of substances of animal origin and of natural substances or concentrates, rose, geranium and so on, to improve or modify the synthetic materials he uses.

Four substances of animal origin, known to perfumers as 'fixatives', have been in use for centuries. Ambergris from the sperm or cachalot whale, castor from the beaver, civet from the civet cat, and musk from the musk deer.

I. AMBERGRIS

This is formed in a lump or series of lumps in the stomach or intestines of the sperm whale, *Physeter catodon*. How or why it is formed is not precisely known but it occurs only rarely. The whale's food is chiefly squid, cuttle fish or octopus and it is possible that the indigestible mandibles of the cuttle fish, nearly always seen in lumps of ambergris, give rise to the formation of this amorphous material, varying in size from a few ounces to a hundredweight or more. Much of it has come from seaports in the Indian ocean. So valuable was it from the fifteenth century onwards that fortunes were made from favourable finds, either those thrown up on the sea shore or by securing a whale that contained the substance. Large lumps are now extremely rare and an authenticated specimen sold in London in 1913 weighing 336 pounds, was by all accounts exceptional.

Ambergris lumps are smooth and polished, light in weight, and they vary in colour from silver grey to golden or dark brown to black. The black is the least valuable. Ambergris in the lump has no strong aromatic odour but its property of fixing other perfumes makes it extremely valuable. Indeed it has been said that while a scent fixed with musk will last for days, one fixed with ambergris will last months. In the 1950s the best kind sold for £6 an ounce (£212 kg.).[1]

The name 'amber' or 'ambre' was often used to describe ambergris

---

[1] Bovill, E. W., 'Musk & Amber', *Notes & Queries* 1953, CXCVIII (Reprint, 9.)

during the sixteenth and seventeenth centuries.[2] Pomanders in use during that period, though containing ambergris usually had additional stronger aromatic substances to give them a distinctive scent. Though ambergris is now used less than formerly, one method is to make an extract by powdering a piece and adding alcohol; the mixture is then shaken for several days and filtered. A noted cosmetic chemist wrote: 'it imparts a velvetness to fine perfumes, unobtainable with any other raw material'.[3] An artificial ambergris is now obtainable.

2. CASTOR (OR CASTOREUM)

This is the name given to the dried preputial follicles of the beaver, *Castor fiber*. The beaver is indigenous to Canada and Western Russia. The glands, 2 to 3 inches long, and known as 'pods', contain a whitish substance which becomes a glossy reddish brown when dry. The characteristic odour is due to a volatile oil. The substance is made into a tincture for use in perfume.

3. CIVET

Of the two species, *Viverra civetta* and *V. zibetha*, the former, from Abysinnia or other mountainous ranges of Africa, is said to yield the better civet. This is obtained from the anal pouches of the civet cat, an animal about three feet in length, ash coloured and black spotted, having a tail which is black and ringed towards its end, of less length than the body. It has two black bands round the throat and one round its face. A mane runs the whole length of its spine and the tail bristles up at will. The civet material of commerce is much like a glazed yellowish brown pomade, having a distinctive odour, obnoxious when first obtained but very pleasant and attractive when sufficiently diluted. It is generally used as a strong tincture. The 'absolute', made from the raw material is costly,

---

[2] 'Tell me if thou canst (and truly) whence doth come
This *Camphire, Storax, Spiknard, Galbanum;*
These *Musks*, these *Ambers*, and those other smells
(Sweet as the Vestrie of the Oracles.)' (Robert Herrick, 1648, O.U.P. Reprint, 1921, 156.)

[3] Poucher, *op. cit.*, I, 304.

about £375 a kilogramme. Civet was formerly imported in large ox horns. Civet was used at one time by the Italians for perfuming gloves. An indication of the esteem in which civet was held by perfumers in the sixteenth and seventeenth centuries is the large number of signboards, billheads and trade cards which bore a representation of the civet cat. The sign continued in use into the nineteenth century. Kendall & Son, for example, used this name at 447 West Strand, London, as late as 1816 and they advertised their eight branches of the 'Civet Catt', widely dispersed from Liverpool to Brighton. Thomas Overton of New Bond Street, London, informed his patrons that he was to be found at 'The Civet Cat and Rose'.

The use of civet was widely known and listeners to *Much Ado about Nothing* would have appreciated Pedro's remark, speaking of Benedick: 'Nay, a' rubs himself with civet: can you smell him out by that?' whereupon Claudio comments: 'That's as much as to say, the sweet youth's in Love'. (Act III, sc. ii)

4. MUSK

This name is given to the dark brown grains, much like moist gingerbread, taken from the pod, the size of a large walnut, of the male musk deer, *Moschus moschiferus*. Musk was first mentioned in Europe by St Jerome in the fourth century AD. Both musk and the musk deer were accurately described by Marco Polo on his return from China in the late thirteenth century.[4] He told how hunters in the Shansi province of China took the membrane or sac from the male musk deer. Only the male has this pod but as the male cannot be readily distinguished at a distance from the female, many musk deer have been slaughtered to no purpose. Even in Marco Polo's day the pods were valuable and as Western Europe became more luxury minded in its demands for perfumes and for its use in medicines so did the price of musk pods increase, particularly when Cairo became the great centre for its distribution. So highly prized was this commodity that soon after the East India Company obtained its charter from Queen Elizabeth I in 1600, it was laid down that no servant of the Company was to trade in musk—the profits of musk trading were to be for the Company. At that period musk pods were being sold for over £2

---

[4] 'Its coat is like the larger kind of deer, its feet and tail are those of the antelope but it has not the horns. It is provided with four projecting teeth or tusks . . .' *The Travels of Marco Polo the Venetian*, Everyman ed. London, 1925, 137–8.

an ounce. The price of musk is now about £750 per pound. Not only was musk used in perfumes and flavourings but in the Tudor period it was a favourite perfume for the lozenges enjoyed as sweetmeats. It was also an ingredient in many compound preparations in the sixteenth and seventeenth century pharmacopoeias and had a reputation for relieving melancholy.

For use, the hair and hide are cut away from the pod. The pods were exported in boxes known as musk caddies.(17) (18). The pleasing odour develops when the pod is dried and subsequently soaked in water. It has then a subtle odour and a diffusive power. Artificial musks of complicated formulae have been devised: these are known as 'musk ambrettes'.

The Perfume Industry of Grasse

The ancient hillside town of Grasse in the Maritime Alps of France, eleven miles north of Cannes on the famous Route Napoléon, is known throughout the world as the centre of the perfume industry. The perfumery houses invite visitors to see something of the processes described below. Fortunate are those who arrive when a whole floor is covered with jonquils, roses or tuberose. The visitor will see modern equipment but here and there he will find some older copper, pear-shaped alembics, more than a metre in height, still being used for distilling.(23)

The earliest writer to comment upon the Grasse flower industry was Papon in 1787. He said that the orange, citron and Spanish jasmine all gave the air a delicious perfume. At that period Grasse was also noted for its tanneries and for glove making, green and red gloves being particularly mentioned. It was about this time too that the perfumers were superceding the former Gantiers-parfumeurs. One of the last of these was Francois Fragonard, father of the celebrated artist, J. H. Fragonard. The Fragonard home in Grasse, decorated with murals by the artist, is to become an Arts Centre. During the artist's boyhood the making of perfumed rosewater was a speciality of Grasse and it has been suggested by Boyer that this may have influenced the young artist in his many paintings of roses.[5]

In the early part of the nineteenth century the cultivation of plants for perfumery was in the hands of small farmers, some of whom distilled

---

[5] Boyer, Dr Jean, *La France et Ses Parfums*, Paris, 1960–1, *III*, 30.

their oils by rudimentary apparatus, selling the products to the manu-facturing houses. By 1898 larger-scale processing became general and the manufacturers formed a Syndicat des Parfumeurs-Distillateurs des Alpes Maritimes. This, in 1941, led to a wider participation in what is now known as the Groupement Interprofessionel des Fleurs et Plantes de la region de Grasse. Fractional distillation was first applied to perfume pro-duction in 1841. Extraction of the essential oils from flowers by using volatile solvents started in 1856 and finally, towards the end of the nine-teenth century, the great advances in synthetic chemistry enabled per-fumes to be enriched by artificially prepared substances and thereby enlarged the scope of the artist-perfumer.

Almost the whole year round flowers bloom in an agreeable climate, the violet from January to March; mimosa in February, huge sprays of yellow blossoms on trees 30 to 40 feet high; the jonquil from February to April; rose and orange in May; jasmine, white and full of odour, and tuberose from July to August; and in the autumn rosemary, cherry laurel and bushy plants such as lavender, clary sage, brooms and mints. In addition to preparing the essential oils from all these, Grasse manufac-turers also process imported materials like citronella from China and patchouli leaves from Java-Sumatra in order to provide a complete range of natural oils and essences. The production of oils from almonds and from walnuts is also undertaken.

In the Garrigues, the name given to the million or more acres of lime-stone uplands between the Cevennes and the Mediterranean, grow thyme, lavender, juniper and rosemary. The larger kind of lavender, commonly known as 'aspic' is best suited to the Herault province, hot in summer and cold in winter.

Some idea of the enormous quantities of flowers and plants handled by the Grasse manufacturers can be gained from the annual reports of the industry, for example: roses 370 tons, narcissi 175 tons, violet leaves 270 tons, lavender and lavandin 56,000 tons, and so on. Cultivation is still in small plots, not in immense fields, and the growers bring their crops direct to the distillers for processing.

Methods of preparing the basic floral or natural oils

These are chiefly three—distillation, expression and extraction.

[44]

DISTILLATION

It was Paracelsus (1493–1541), physician and chemist, who developed the new laboratory techniques for the preparation of his new chemical medicines and for the distillation of what were called essential oils, i.e. volatile oils, from plants. These he described as 'quintessences'. Distillation has been the means principally used for plants, barks, woods, and for some flowers. Flowers such as lavender may be suspended on frames in the still; steam is passed through and the essential oil contained in the flower heads is collected. The lower aqueous layers may be used for toilet waters.

EXPRESSION

This term is applied to the method of grating the rind of fruits such as lemons, collecting the oil in a sponge and subsequently refining it. The method has been held to give a better finished product than by distilling the rinds. Mechanical means are also adopted for the grating process. Another method is to crush the whole fruit, then to spray the mass and extract the oil by centrifuge.

MACERATION AND ABSORPTION

Various methods were devised during the nineteenth century. These were based upon the principle that there was a chemical affinity between the aroma constituent of the flowers and a fatty substance. By absorbing the scented oils in the fat and then treating the fat with alcohol, the aromatic oil could be extracted. An alternative method attributed to a French chemist, Millon, was to percolate flowers with ether or other suitable solvent. This produced a solid waxy mass possessing the scent of the flower in its purest and most concentrated form. These solids came to be called 'concrete essences' or merely 'concretes'. If these concretes are extracted with alcohol so that the waxes are removed, the resulting solution of the aromatic constituents is described as an 'absolute'. It is correspondingly priced. Synthetic substances can be added to these absolutes to form new compound absolutes.

[45]

ENFLEURAGE

This was an absorption process whereby flowers were spread on greased plates, the flowers being frequently removed so that more and more perfume could be absorbed by the grease or fat. For the more delicate aromas of flowers like jasmine and tuberose this method could be carried out without heat. Modification of this by spreading the flowers on fine net between glass frames was introduced by two French perfumers, D. Sémeris of Nice and L. T. Piver of Paris. In recent years the enfleurage process has become too costly to be continued. New solvents have been brought into use: these extract the oils from delicately perfumed flowers without impairing the aroma.

ADSORPTION

Various patents have been granted for adsorption methods of obtaining oils from flowers where normal distillation is less effective. Air or gases are passed over the flowers and these, containing the odour, are then passed over charcoal which adsorbs it; finally this odorous material is subjected to steam which carries off the perfumed oil. Alternatives to the activated charcoal are kaolin, clay or colloidal silicon. These general methods are said to produce better results and to be cheaper in operation.[6]

Some of the principal materials used in perfumes (20)

Aloe Wood. The resinous wood, oriental lignaloes, is from the tree, *Aquilaria agalloche*, grown in Assam, Bengal, Burma and Java. It has been recorded from the time of the Egyptians and the Biblical references also suggest it was this wood which was used as incense. The highly perfumed wood is distilled.

Benzoin. A resinous gum from the tree, *Styrax benzoin*, chiefly from Java and Siam. When it was first described in the fourteenth century by Ibn Batuta, the traveller who found it growing in Sumatra, it was called 'Java frankincense'. It was so well reputed in the Middle Ages that quantities were included as presents to the doges of Venice in 1461 and 1490. It was imported into England from Siam in 1635.[7] The gum was used

---

[6] Moncrieff, C. W., *The Chemical Senses*, London, 1967, 604–5.

[7] Flückiger, F. A. & Hanbury, Daniel, *Pharmacographia*, London, 1874, 362.

as incense by the Greek Church. It gives 'body' to most types of perfume.

Bergamot oil. From the fresh peel of the greenish orange-like fruit of *Citrus bergamia* grown in Calabria. The skins are first pierced and the oil collected and filtered. The industry is in the hands of an official Consortium. About 400 tons of fruit are produced annually. The oil was first used in perfumes at the beginning of the eighteenth century.

Bois de Rose oil. This oil, from various trees in French Guiana and northern Brazil, has come into prominence during this century as a useful source of linalol, the scent associated with honeysuckle, lilac and lily perfumes.

Broom flowers. Because of its honey-scented flowers the broom is cultivated in Provence. The flowers are used to make a concentrated essence.

Calamus oil. Distilled from the rhizome of the sweet flag, *Acorus calamus*. The plant is grown in Europe and in the USA. The oil is particularly liked in India.

Citronella oil. Various grasses native to Java and Ceylon, when distilled, yield this oil. The industry is on a large scale, chiefly because of the heavy demand for the oil from the soap makers.

Clary Sage oil. Clary sage was first used as a medicine in England in the seventeenth century when it was recommended to be fried with eggs. The flowering tops of *Salvia sclarea* are used to obtain an oil which has a distinctive aroma. The Mediterranean region is the chief source. Poucher says this sage is used in some varieties of vermouth as a flavouring.[8]

Chypre. The name usually denotes a heavy clinging type of perfume.

Frankincense (or Olibanum). This milky gum-resin is exuded from various species of *Boswellia* trees. Excisions are made in the bark and the exudate when dry is harvested in the form of translucent lumps or tears. According to reports the method of collection has changed little during the past 2,000 years. The principal source is Dhofar, a province of Arabia, though some comes from East Africa. Frankincense was used by the Egyptians as early as the seventeenth century BC, as indicated by illustrations of both trees and bags of gum in paintings of that period. Its modern use in perfumery is mainly as a fixative in scents, especially of the heavy oriental type and in face powders. Like myrrh, frankincense is one of the traditional Epiphany offerings.

Geranium oil. Distilled from the leaves of various kinds of geraniums (pelargoniums), grown in Algeria, in France from the middle of the nine-

---

[8] Poucher, *op. cit.*, II, 129.

teenth century, in Bulgaria and Spain. The rose odour makes it an accepted basis of many artificial floral oils of the rose type and it is of great use to the soap makers.

Jasmine. From many kinds of jasmine flowers, chiefly from India where the perfume is highly esteemed and from Grasse. The former spelling was 'jessamine'.

Labdanum. Obtained from different kinds of rock rose, e.g. *Cistus landaisperus* and *C. labdonum*, grown in the countries bordering the Mediterranean and particularly round the Esterel mountains of Provence. It is a sticky balsam employed as a fixative and has the odour of ambergris.

Lavender oil. Two varieties of lavender, *Lavendula vera*, are grown commercially in England—the Giant Blue and the Dwarf Munstead. The oil is distilled from the flowering heads. French perfumers rely largely upon oil from the wild lavenders of Provence. Spike Lavender oil from *L. spica*, grown in France and Spain, provides an oil used in the soap industry.

Lemon grass oil. Distilled from two kinds of lemon grass indigenous to S. India and Malaya. The oil yields ionone, a constituent of all violet based perfumes.

Macassar oil. True macassar oil, of butter-like consistency, is produced by crushing the seeds of a plant, *Schleichera trijuga*, grown in the East Indies. Macassar oil was much used in a hair pomade fashionable during the nineteenth century.

Morse powder. This powder was made by grinding walrus tusks. It was almost a monopoly of two companies in Bordeaux. Formerly used by the French cosmetic industry for rouge and face powder, it has been superseded by other ingredients, making it unnecessary to slaughter walruses for this purpose.

Myrrh. Myrrh was in use as a perfume, as a preservative, and as an ingredient in incense from early times. It was known and used by Egyptians, Hebrews and Arabs. Two kinds have been employed—the true myrrh (herrabol myrrh) and perfumed or sweet myrrh, also called bdellium or opoponax. Opoponax perfume was an Edwardian favourite. Both kinds are collected as exudations in the form of pale yellow or yellowish-brown lumps from small trees in Arabia, Abysinnia or Somaliland. Myrrh was one of the three customary royal offerings at Epiphany, the observance of which goes back to the time of Edward I. Traditionally it was one of the gifts brought by the Three Wise Men from the East. The use of myrrh for medicinal purposes continued into the middle of this century.

Oakmoss resin. Surprisingly useful materials for perfumery can be extracted from such unlikely sources as the lichens from trees like the oak and pine. Oakmoss resin is a part of the industry's raw material. Bulgaria offers concentrates of oakmoss and of various kinds of pine trees, juniper and the like.

Olibanum. See the note under Frankincense above.

Orange flower oil (Neroli oil). This is distilled from the fresh flowers of the sweet orange. The orange is said to have been brought from the East by Portuguese traders in the fifteenth century, hoping to cultivate it in the Iberian peninsula. Orange flowers were used as perfume in the seventeenth century. Writing in 1691, W. Salmon reported that the Water made with them is not only a good perfume but as a remedy prevented and helped fevers.[9] The seeds (pips) he said, killed worms, resisted poisons and helped scorpion stings. A synthetic compound resembling orange flower oil is available. Other varieties of orange flower oils are bigarade oil from the bitter orange tree, petitgrain mandarin oil from the leaves and twigs of the mandarin orange tree, and a petitgrain oil from the leaves of the bitter orange tree grown either in France, Sicily and Spain or in Paraguay. The alternative name of Neroli for orange flower oil has as its derivation its use in the 1670s by the second wife of the Prince of Neroli, Flavio Orsini, for perfuming gloves, thereafter called Guanti de Neroli.[10]

Orris. The rhizome of the pale-flowered iris, *Iris pallida*, from Tuscany is much used in sachets, soaps and violet powders.

Otto of Rose. For more than two thousand years the rose has been the choicest of flowers in the Near East and in Europe. Poets have sung its praise, the Romans could hardly have enough of it, sprinkling their food with its perfume or with its petals, and Cleopatra is said to have laid a carpet of roses when she sought to win back the fickle Antony. Persian poets of the thirteenth and fourteenth centuries, Saidi in *Gulistan* or The Garden of Roses, and Hafiz, found in the rose new intensities of fragrance. The process of distilling rose water was known in Persia in the ninth century if the report be true that the Caliph Al Ma'mun (813–33) could insist upon a tribute of 30,000 phials a year from the Shiraz district.[11]

---

9 Salmon, W., *op. cit.* 119a, 143a.

10 Flückiger & Hanbury, *op. cit.* 113.

11 Holmyard, *op. cit.* 49. Holmyard describes the type of apparatus mentioned by Geber in the ninth century and he reproduces an illustration of it from *Die Alchemie des Geber* by E. Darmstetter, Springer-Verlag, Berlin.

The extreme delicacy of otto (or attar) of rose seems to have become appreciated in the early part of the seventeenth century when production started at Shiraz. From Persia cultivation of the rose and production of the otto spread to India, N. Africa and Turkey.

Over 250 years ago the Turks introduced rose cultivation into Bulgaria, then part of the Ottoman Empire. The first Bulgarian traders filled their saddle bags with bottles of the otto and rode through Europe to sell them. This led to a flourishing undertaking in an area now extending for many miles and which has the name of Valley of Roses. At the height of the flowering season in May, the scent of roses carries for miles. This is true also for the orange groves whether in Bulgaria, Spain or in Southern France. At first the Bulgarian growers distilled their own otto in hooded copper vessels called 'alembics'.(19, 23) For the past 70 years, large-scale manufacture has needed modern equipment and the industry is now controlled by State organizations.(21) It takes 3,500 kilogrammes weight of roses (over $3\frac{1}{2}$ tons) to produce 1 kilo (2.2 lb.) of otto, the value of which may be as high as £600 (or £15 an ounce), depending upon the variety of rose from which the otto is distilled. Rose otto is shipped in sealed drums, known as 'konkouns', decorated with ribbons in the national colours.(24) Bulgaria prides herself upon her red rose otto from *Rosa damascena* but additionally makes rose concrete and rose absolute.

It was thought at one time that similarity of climate and of soils in Russia to those of Bulgaria might provide opportunity for successful otto production in Russia. Experiments so far have not proved commercially successful.[12]

At Grasse many varieties of roses are distilled, including the white and the cabbage rose, *Rosa centifolia*. A rose geranium oil is also prepared by distilling geranium oil over fresh rose petals.

Patchouli oil. This is distilled from the dried leaves of the patchouli plant (*Pogostemon patchouli*) and similar plants grown in India and the East Indies (Java-Sumatra). The oil was formerly used for perfuming Indian shawls.[13] Patchouli perfume was much used during the Edwardian period.

Peau d'Espagne. The name given to perfumed leather prepared in Spain. It was also encased in sachets for perfuming gloves. Philip Massinger refers to perfumed leather in two of his plays: 'Sweet Madam, keep your gloves to your nose. Or let me fetch some perfumes . . .' and 'Where are my

---

[12] Newman, Bernard, *Bulgarian Background*, London, 1961, 67–8.
[13] Poucher, *op. cit.* II, 322.

shoes? . . . Those that your Ladyship gave order should be made of the Spanish perfumed skins?'[14]

Rosemary oil. Used in blending in perfumes such as Eau de Cologne. Both French and English oils are available.

Sandalwood oil. Chiefly from Mysore, India, where the heart wood and the roots of the evergreen tree, *Santalum album*, are distilled. Another more recent source for this oil is Western Australia.

Synthetics. The general name applied to a host of chemical compounds used in the perfumery industry for blending with naturally produced oils or essences and for making artificial perfumes resembling those made from the natural oils. Some compounds are derived from natural oils, such as ionone, having a violet odour, from lemon grass oil though this may also be made chemically. In the 1920s new chemical compounds, the aldehydes, were made; these, unstable in nature, were then at the disposal of laboratories for still further additions to the range of the synthetics previously existing.

Tuberose. The tuberose, *Polyanthes tuberosa*, produces white flowers, slightly pinkish on the outside, on long stalks. The flowers are grown from tubers. Whether in France or in India the flower has a most insidious and intense scent. Volatile solvents are used to extract the delicate perfume.

Vanilla. The only orchid, *Vanilla fragrans*, to be cultivated on an industrial scale. The Belgian botanist, Morren, took seed from the Museum of Paris about 1822 and began to grow it in Madagascar. The pod or bean is used. Essences from it are often used in cooking.

Nature's own Perfumes

Attempts have been made over the years to capture the natural scents of the countryside. Two of these, New Mown Hay and Jockey Club, appeared in the nineteenth century; the third, Earth Perfume, has been available only a few years.

NEW MOWN HAY

The peculiarly attractive odour arising from a newly cut hay crop is

---

[14] Massinger, Philip (1573-1638), *A New Way to Pay Old Debts*, 1633, Act I sc. iii; *The City Madam*, 1632, Act I, sc. i.

known to everyone. This is due especially to the sweet-scented vernal grass, one of the grasses normally growing in a hay field. Chemists have found that the chemical substance responsible for the distinctive odour of new mown hay is coumarin, identified by W. H. Perkin, the dye chemist. This is the basis of the artificial perfume made to resemble the actual scent of the new mown hay. Formerly well liked, it is little in fashion now.

Jockey Club

This name, like New Mown Hay, reflects the choice of fragrant country smells. Jockey Club perfume was intended to reproduce the fragrance of Epsom Downs in the late Spring. Various bouquets were sold under this name.

Earth Perfume (Matti ka Attar)

The characteristic odour associated with fresh rain is not the rain itself but arises from clays, rocks, and soils after exposure to sunshine when they are moistened with rain. Not only man but animals react to this odour. Septimus Piesse, a French perfumer who migrated to London and who set up a Laboratory of Flowers, was probably the first to call attention to the refreshing odour arising when earth, clay or chalk was moistened with rain. He was of opinion that it was because of the inherent qualities of the substances themselves and not to those contained in the rain or water. He had himself experimented with distilled water and reported he found the odour every bit as pronounced.

Perfume has been made from this unexpected source. A perfumery at Kannauj, near Lucknow, India, offers 'Matti ka attar' (Earth perfume), made by distilling the vapours that arise during the rainy season from disks of clay previously exposed to the hot sun. These disks are distilled by steam and the oily vapours that arise are absorbed in sandalwood oil. The resulting 'earth perfume' is called 'Matti ka attar'. Two laboratory workers in Melbourne, Australia, have used various rocks and clays, exposed to the sun and then moistened with rain or water, to find out what chemical constituents make up this distinctive smell. This 'argillaceous odour', arising from the rocks, clays, etc., is now found to be caused by the contaminants of the atmosphere, i.e. volatile decomposed matter from

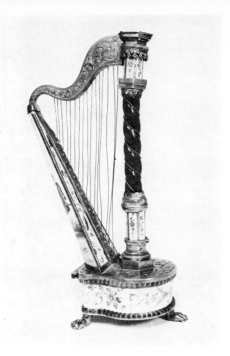
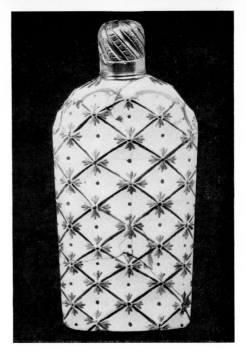
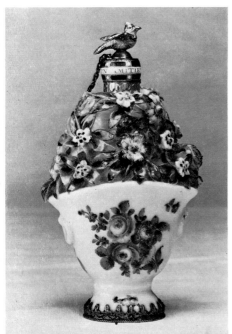
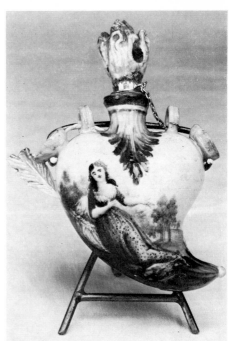

44. (*top, left*) PORCELAIN SCENT BOTTLE IN THE FORM OF *A HARP*
Stem enamelled in blue and floral decoration and pastoral scenes. Probably French, 18th century. (Wellcome Institute of the History of Medicine)

45. (*top, right*) SCENT BOTTLE, FRENCH, 18TH CENTURY
Enamelled in bright pink and gold with gold stopper. (Wellcome Institute of the History of Medicine)

46. (*below, left*) SCENT BOTTLE, DRESDEN, 18TH CENTURY
Biconical, vase in two parts, the lower white, decorated with roses, the upper of brilliantly coloured flowers and foliage. The inscription 'Gage de mon amitié' on the enamelled collar surmounted by a bird. (Leon Givaudan Collection. Photo: Raoul Foulon, Paris)

47. (*below, right*) SCENT BOTTLE, 18TH CENTURY
Probably Vienna. Heart shape decorated with a figure at the base. Two rings for suspension. The arrow in relief, the stopper a flower fastened to the bottle by a tiny chain. (Leon Givaudan Collection)

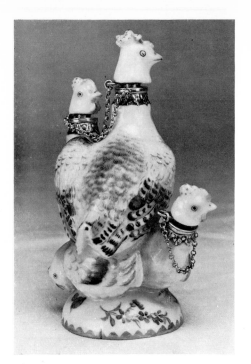

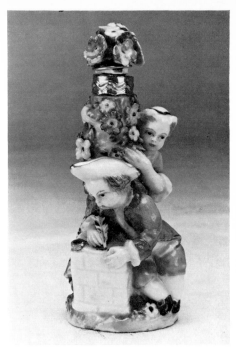

48. *SCENT BOTTLE, CHELSEA, 18TH CENTURY*
Three bottles in one, each a chicken, the heads surmount gold chased stoppers: a fourth chicken at the base. (Leon Givaudan Collection. Photo: Raoul Foulon, Paris)

49. *SCENT BOTTLE, CHELSEA. 18TH CENTURY*
A notary public writing a letter for the girl clinging to a flower covered tree which forms the bottle. The gold stopper surmounted by flower petals. (Leon Givaudan Collection. Photo: Raoul Foulon, Paris)

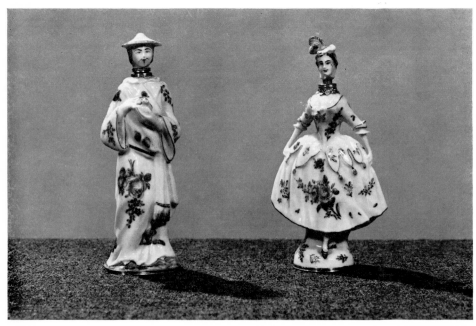

50. *SCENT BOTTLES IN THE FORM OF FIGURINES, CHELSEA, 18TH CENTURY*
Left: Chinaman. Right: Dancing lady—both 10 cm. (Schreiber Collection, Victoria & Albert Museum. Crown Copyright)

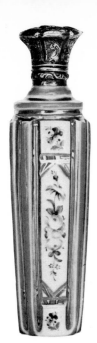

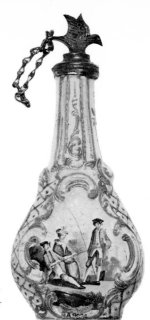

51. (left) SCENT BOTTLE, CHELSEA, 18TH CENTURY
Decorated with floral panels; silver stopper. (London Museum)

52. (right) SCENT BOTTLE, CHELSEA, 18TH CENTURY
Enamelled, gold decoration with coloured figures in a fishing scene, the stopper in the form of a dove. (London Museum)

53. (below) VINAIGRETTE IN GOLD AND ENAMEL
Basin shaped, richly decorated, with chain attachment and pearl ornamentation. (Wellcome Institute of the History of Medicine)

54. (bottom of page) VINAIGRETTE IN GOLD AND ENAMEL
Egg shaped, with heavy decoration of flowers and birds. (Wellcome Institute of the History of Medicine)

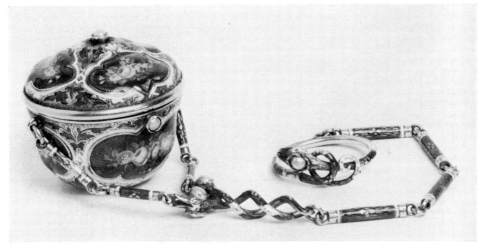

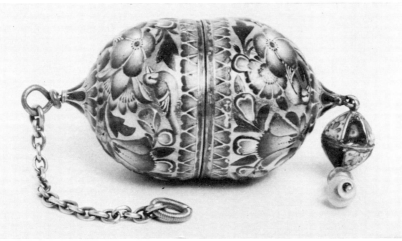

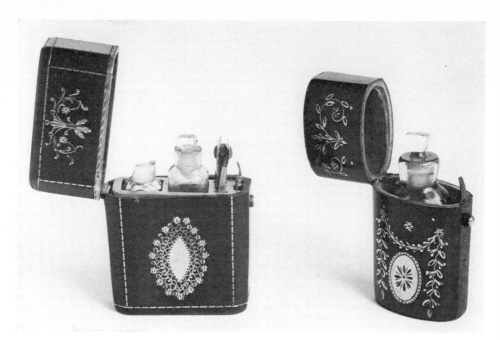

55. TORTOISESHELL PERFUME CASES WITH PIQUE DECORATION, 18TH CENTURY
Each contains glass stoppered bottles. Height 5 cm. (Private Collection)

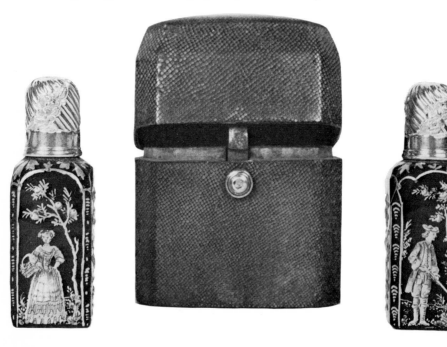

56. SCENT BOTTLE CASE IN SHAGREEN, c. 1770
Velvet lined for two glass bottles in blue with figures and floral sprays in gilt. Gilded covers to stoppers.
Probably London make. Height 6.75 cm.

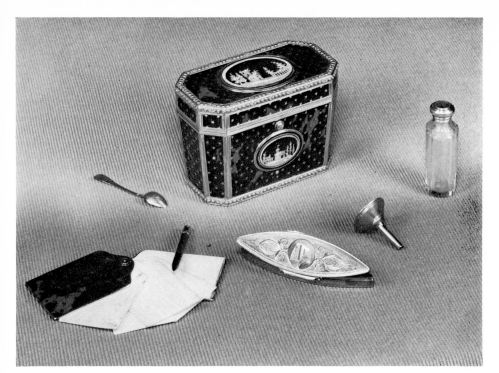

57. (*above*) FRENCH
PERFUME COFFRET,
LATE 18TH CENTURY
*Tortoiseshell encrusted with
gold decorated with Italian
country scenes, fitted with a
glass bottle, funnel, spoon,
patch box and writing tablet.
(Leon Givaudan Collection.
Photo: Raoul   Foulon,
Paris)*

58. (*right*) TOILET
WATER CASE, MID-
18TH CENTURY
*Made for Princess Sophia.
Decorated lid. Two diamond
cut bottles, capped with silver with monogram S. Height
of bottles 8 cm. (London
Museum)*

59. ENGLISH EARTHEN-
WARE JARS, PROB-
ABLY FOR COSMETICS,
LATE 17TH CENTURY
*Globular-shaped, decorated
with rows of alternate blue
and mauve spots, pink tinted
glaze. (Wellcome Institute
of the History of Medicine)*

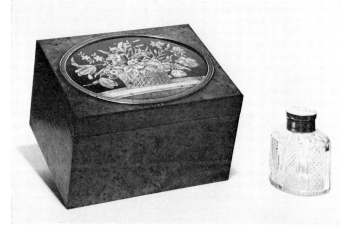

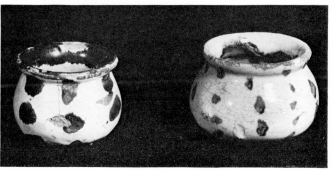

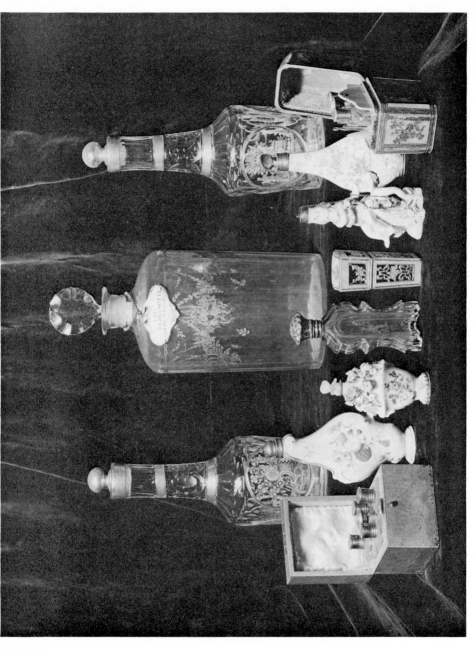

60. *FLACONS AND PERFUME CASES, 18TH and 19TH CENTURIES*

Top, centre: decanter with medallion EAU BERGAMOTTE HOUBIGANT A PARIS. Below, left and right: Two fitted cases, sbagreen and porcelain. (Houbigant Antique Collection, U.S.A.)

61 and 62. COSMETIC JAR & BILL, BARTHO VALLE &
BROTHER, LONDON, 1771
Items are Florence Water, Naples Soap & pot, Lavender and Hungary
(Water); the cosmetic jar, delftware, shows Valle at 21 Haymarket.
(Historical Collection: Pharmaceutical Society of Great Britain)

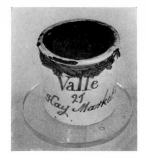

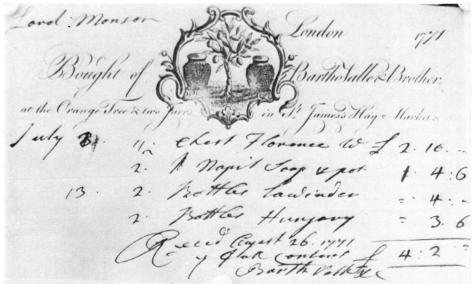

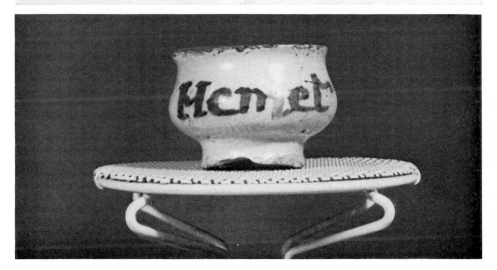

63. DELFTWARE POT, HAMET, LONDON, 18TH CENTURY
(Historical Collection: Pharmaceutical Society of Great Britain)

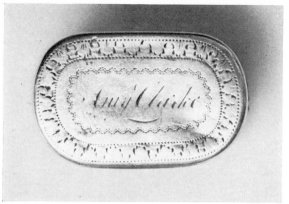

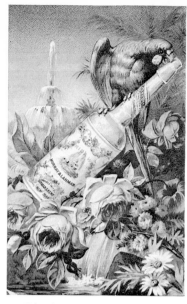

64. PATCH BOX, SILVER, 19TH CENTURY
Engraved, with name 'Amy Clarke'. Possibly of Bilston manufacture. (*Wellcome Institute of the History of Medicine*)
66. (*below*) POT LIDS—BEARS AND BEARS' GREASE, 19TH CENTURY
Top: Bear on pole; Bear and keeper snowballed. Centre: Bears in wood, rare; Below left: Patey & Co., Lombard Street, London (*black on white ground*). Below right: Whitaker & Co., 69 Hatton Garden, London (*polychrome*)

65. (*above*) ADVERTISING CARD, USA, LATE 19TH CENTURY
Murray & Lanman Florida Water

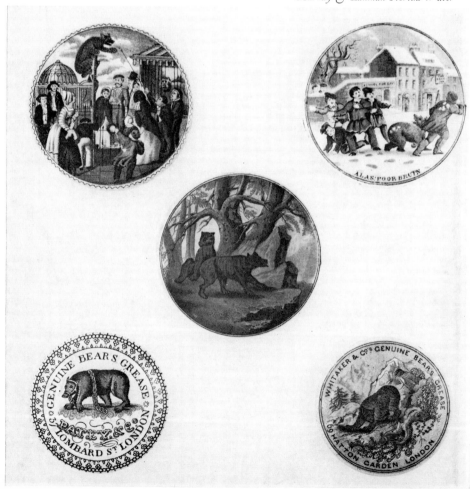

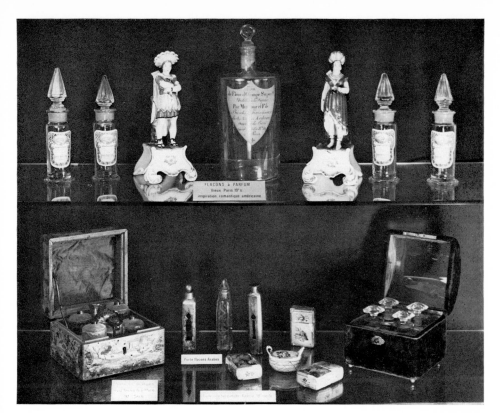

67. (above) PERFUME FLACONS
AND CASES, 19TH CENTURY
Upper row: Made in Paris, the figures in
American Indian style. Lower row: centre,
metal cases for Arab perfumes. (Musée
Fragonard, Grasse)

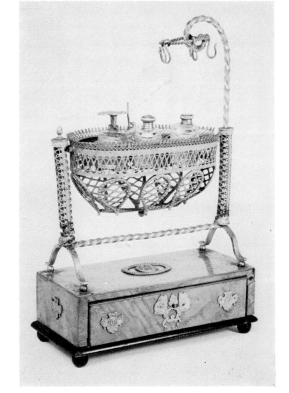

68. (right) CRADLE SCENT BOTTLE
HOLDER, LATE 18TH CENTURY
Gilt filigree, with bottles and stand and
drawer below. (Wellcome Institute of the
History of Medicine)

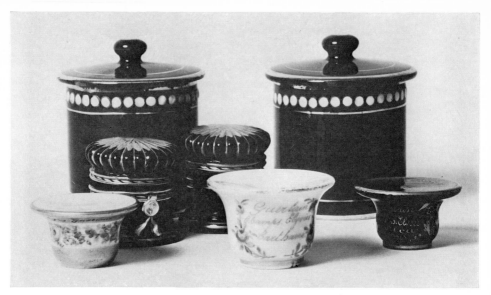

69. (*above*) PORCELAIN COSMETIC JARS AND ROUGE POTS, FRENCH, MID-19TH CENTURY
Decorated in Second Empire style, the smaller dark blue jars with metal mounts. The rouge pots have flat covers. (Guerlain Collection, Paris)

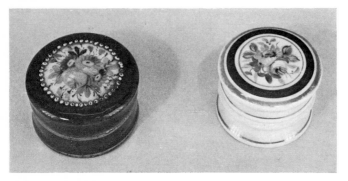

70. (*left*) COSMETIC JARS, PORCELAIN, 19TH CENTURY
Height 3.5 cm. (Historical Collection: Pharmaceutical Society of Great Britain)

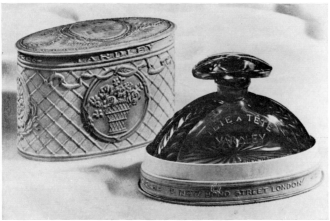

71. CRYSTAL PERFUME BOTTLE AND CASE, 1921
Designed for Yardley's Tete-a-Tete perfume. Case reproduces an ancient ivory casket.

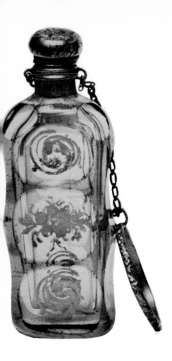

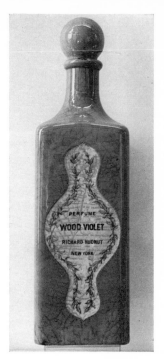

72. (left) SCENT BOTTLE,
GLASS, 19TH CENTURY
*Indented panels with gold decoration
and guard ring. Height 7 cm.
(Wellcome Institute of the History
of Medicine)*

74. (right) PERFUME BOTTLE,
U.S.A., c. 1900
*Violet coloured glass with reserved
panel. (Historical Collection:
Pharmaceutical Society of Great
Britain)*

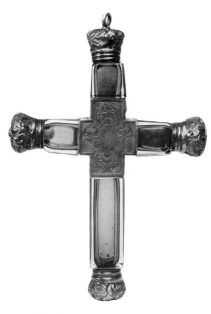

73. CRUCIFORM SCENT BOTTLE, 19TH
CENTURY
*Red Glass, silver mounts and engraved joining
plates. Height 7 cm. (Wellcome Institute of the
History of Medicine)*

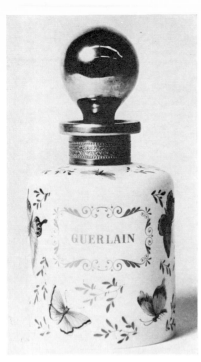

75. (left) OPALINE GLASS PERFUME BOTTLE, GUERLAIN, FRENCH, MID-19TH CENTURY
Decorated with sprigs and butterflies, Second Empire period. (Guerlain Collection, Paris)

76. (right) SCENT BOTTLE WITH MEDALLION OF THE PRINCE REGENT, c. 1820
Probably by Apsley Pellatt. Cut mushroom stopper has portrait of girl. Height 10 cm. (London Museum)

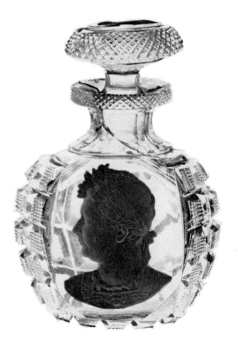

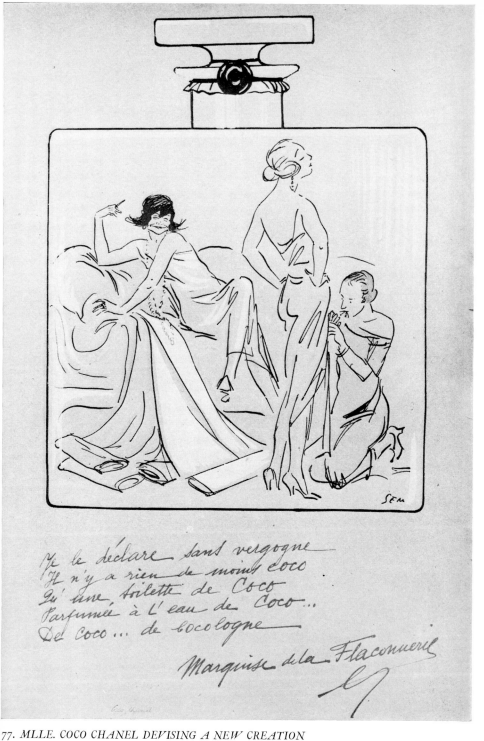

Je le déclare sans vergogne
Il n'y a rien de moins coco
Qu'une toilette de Coco
Parfumée à l'eau de Coco...
De Coco... de cocologne

Marquise de la Flaconnerie

77. MLLE. COCO CHANEL DEVISING A NEW CREATION
Sketch by SEM, c. 1924
The bottle just designed for Chanel No. 5.
'There's nothing less like Coco than a toilette by Coco, perfumed with Cocologne'
Original in the Musée de Périgord, Périgueux. (Photo: R. Gautier & Fils, Périgueux)

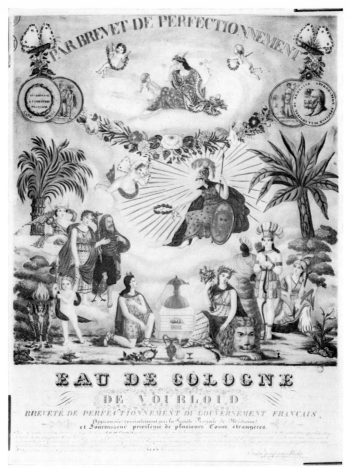

78a. (above) EAU DE COLOGNE SHOWCARD—VOUR-LOUD, PARIS, c. 1823
As soon as a 'Brevet de Perfectionnement' had been granted,
Vourloud and other perfumers issued cards to announce this.
(Photo: Françoise Foliot, Paris. Bouvet Collection, Paris)

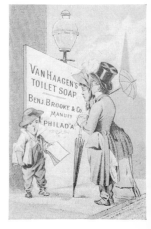

*78b. (right) ADVERTISING CARD, PHILADELPHIA,
LATE 19TH CENTURY*
Van Haagen's Toilet Soap, 10 × 7 cm.

79a. (left) DOUBLE VINAIGRETTE, GLASS, 19TH CENTURY
Metal mounts and foot cavity. (London Museum)
79b. (right) DUCK HEAD SCENT BOTTLE, c. 1880
Pale blue over red glass. Silver stopper. Made by Woodward of Stourbridge. Length 9 cm. (London Museum)

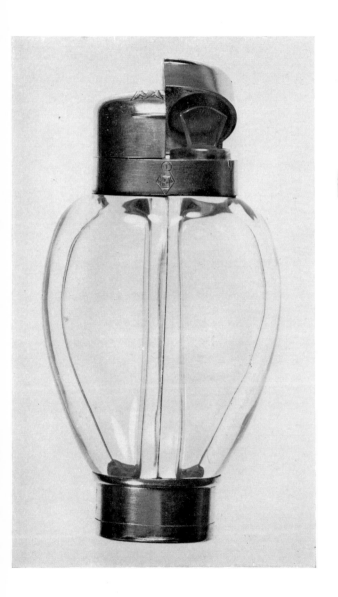

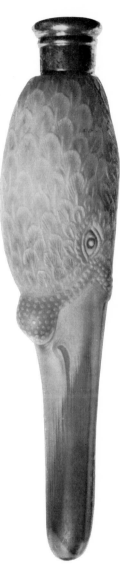

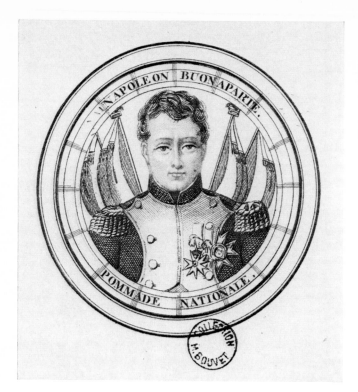

80a. (left) LABEL,
POMMADE NATION-
ALE, LATE 18TH CEN-
TURY
Depicts the young Napoleon.
(Bouvet Collection, Paris)

80b. (right) LABEL, SAVON
DEMARSON, 19TH CENTURY
In colour by Demarson, Chetelat &
Co., Paris (Bouvet Collection,
Paris)

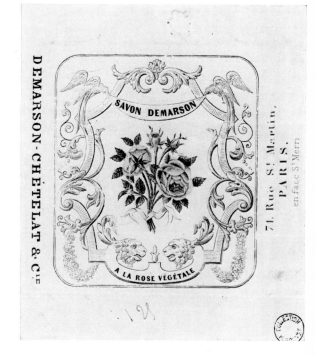

animal and vegetable sources. When the relative humidity of the atmosphere approaches saturation, and rain falls, these contaminants are adsorbed on the earth, clays and rocks. The oil, extracted from these by distillation, is a complex mixture. These workers have suggested the name 'petrichor' for the odour.[15]

[15] Bear, I. J. & Thomas, R. G. (C.S.I.R.O., Melbourne), 'The Nature of Argillaceous Odour, and Genesis of Petrichor', *Nature*, 1964, *201*, 993; *Geochimica et Cosmochimica*, 1966, *30*, 869–79.

{ 6 }

Some Collectable Antiques

IN the earlier chapters some of the antiques associated with perfume have been noted. Here it is proposed to describe under period headings a further variety of antiques which are still collectable.

Sixteenth and Seventeenth centuries

PERFUME CASES

Some of the most elaborate perfume cases for persons of quality were made during the seventeenth century. The Florentine case presented by the Grand Duke of Florence to Oliver, Lord Cromwell, is in black polished wood decorated with marble and inlaid panels. It contains three drawers each holding eight Venetian glass pots covered in fabric embroidered with precious stones.(25) Less spectacular perhaps but of the same period or a little later is a handsome chest almost too richly furnished for a surgeon but nevertheless fitted with his instruments, with ornamental unguent pots all of the same design in relief and with a silver bleeding bowl.(27). This contains the tradition of specially-designed cases for particular uses such as perfumes.

The seaborne trade carried on by the Italians in silks, spices, oils and essences across the Mediterranean encouraged the cities of Italy to furnish the luxuries which their rich merchants demanded. Those monks who were already skilled in chemical processes turned to the arts of distilling and blending floral oils. One of the most enterprising and important, for at least two centuries, was the seventeenth century Fonderia of Santa Maria Novella of Florence, later styled the Officina Profumo-Pharmaceutica, which provided the public with a great variety of perfume oils and essences in narrow bottles, sealed and capped, each with its glass dropper. The bottles were packed in wooden cases in book form. These 'books' were covered in linen or leather, some being finely tooled to resemble typical bindings of the period.(26) The style continued into the eighteenth century.(26, left) It was probably this kind of perfume book that wa given to Samuel Pepys by his nephew (page 20).

Another Fonderia, that of S. Paulina, also of Florence, issued similar book packings of essences bearing the names Flowers of Myrtle, Lemon, Milleflor and Rosemary. The interior of the lid of the book illustrated is decorated with a handsome garden, fountain and trees, with a country gentleman and lady to set off the stately home.(28) These books of per-fumes are scarce and now are rarely seen outside museum collections.

ROSEWATER BOWLS

Silver or silver gilt bowls for use at table for rinsing fingers or more often for refreshing by application of the rosewater to the temple or ears, were customary in large houses and at special functions such as City Company dinners and the Inns of Court, where the practice is still observed. The most likely period in which those in current use were made is the second half of the sixteenth century but those of later periods are regularly offered in the principal sale rooms throughout the country or by specialist dealers. Plain bowls or those with little ornamentation and from 30 to 40 cm. diameter, with wide rims, may give more satisfaction to the pos-sessor than the richly chased and engraved kinds.

CENSERS

When it was customary for the owner of a country mansion to attend divine service in his private chapel he would rarely be satisfied with any-thing less than vessels of the finest workmanship procurable. Many of the vessels used came from the Continent. The silver gilt censer, 20 cm. high, dated about 1600 and engraved in a modern hand 'From the Chapel at Dilston House' is an example of Spanish work. Dilston was the family name of the Earls of Derwentwater. The censer is in three parts, with pierced scrollwork.(29) The sixteenth century Portuguese silver censer, 24.5 cm. high, is of more intricate design, with a buttressed and crocheted spire on a balustrade of columns, with a chain and ornamental inner cover, known as a lily.(30)

SCENT FLAGONS

The Elizabethan scent flagon, London, 1563, height 17 cm., balanced on a slender pedestal, must have added charm to a table graced with a service in silver or silver gilt.(31)

FUMING POTS

While the most usual perfume items of the fifteenth to the seventeenth centuries would have been the pomanders described in Chapter 2, the more humble but necessary fuming pots for cleansing clothes and for fumigating or perfuming rooms should not be overlooked. These, in earthenware, were in almost everyday use from the fifteenth century. The sixteenth century example, 22 cm. high, has wide openings to allow the perfume to diffuse(33); that in brown-green glaze, seventeenth or early eighteenth century and 12 cm. high, has perforations in the upper part and in the rim.(34)

Eighteenth century

For sheer beauty of design and workmanship, the metal work in gold and silver, the exquisite enamelling, the finish of the small fitted perfume cases, all invite admiration, and focus the collector's attention. If he is looking for metal objects he has a wide choice in silver cassolettes or pastille burners, pot-pourri jars, vinaigrettes, scent bottles and fitted cases, patch boxes and cosmetic cases. He may not perhaps light upon a cassolette of the type designed by Robert Adam and made by Matthew Boulton in his new Soho Works near Birmingham in 1779(32) but he may pick up an equally rare and interesting piece like the small iron fumigator illustrated.(35) When pot-pourri became fashionable, Wedgwood made elegant pot-pourri vases in black basalt in the late eighteenth century. These were decorated in 'famille rose' enamels with sprays of flowers in reddish brown. These vases, about 32 cm. in height, with loop handles, had inner covers and pierced domed outer covers. It was during the nineteenth century that there came a flood of pastille burners of quite a different style, the miniature houses made in pottery by the hundreds in Staffordshire, all highly decorated. These are of such diverse style that they have an appeal of their own to collectors of pottery of that period.

VINAIGRETTES

Their use has been described in Chapter 3. Some unusual forms are worth notice, such as that in gold in the form of a rose,(36) the head of which opens to reveal the grid covering the tapered stem; the George III example in silver showing Windsor Castle in high relief(37); the hunting horn in silver, c. 1860(38); the butterfly, enamelled in naturalistic colours, with sides and base in dark and light blue(39, *right*); or the pearl framed, lozenge type in Directoire style at the very end of the century (39, *left*). From time to time the protection against bad airs, miasmas and plague expected by the owner of a vinaigrette was thought insufficient; an amulet was also worn. One vinaigrette which must have afforded the possessor comfort was in the form of a hand, in opaline glass decorated in enamel, 10 cm. high. The thumb of the hand is set between the first and second finger, the usual means of averting ill from the Evil Eye.(40)

SCENT BOTTLES

These were made in great variety, whether in gold, enamel or in the soft porcelain of Chelsea, Dresden, Vincennes (or Sèvres), Vienna or other manufactories.

The first period of great elegance and luxury that Paris knew was that of Louis XIV. It continued until the end of the reign of Louix XVI in 1793. French goldsmiths were masters in handling their material, gold with alloys. They were well supported by the enamellers whose decorative art was superb. Snuff boxes and scent-bottle cases in gold were set with precious or semi-precious stones, the cases being chased in elaborate designs.

Two fine examples of the French Regency period (1715–23) are the baluster scent bottle, chased and enamelled in blue and white with domestic animal scenes,(41) and the other, also with animals, e.g. the fox and the grapes, with a hinged panel in one side revealing the portrait of a gentleman of the period.(42) The gold bottle ornamented with Watteau subjects, Louis XV, shows figures on a cask in an arbour of grape vines. (42, *right*). The English gold bottle, chased and enamelled with a dove over the stopper, has a carnelian base engraved with a man's hand for use as a seal.(42, *left*) Another gold bottle, for suspension by a gold chain embellished with precious stones, is chased and decorated with flowers and birds in enamel; the plaque is similarly decorated.(8) This is probably English of Louis XV period. Later in date is the engraved silver scent bottle of the William & Mary period with its silver chain.(43)

ENAMELLED PORCELAIN SCENT BOTTLES

In 1760 Louis XV purchased the factory already established at Vincennes and he then ordered a new factory to be built at Sèvres: this was to become the leading manufactory of porcelain in Europe. From that time new colours such as *jaune de jonquil*, *bleu du roi* and the famous *rose du Barry* were introduced for the decoration of soft porcelain (*paté tendre*).

The calabash-shaped bottle, probably French, and late in the century, is enamelled in green and ornamented with flowers in gold, the porcelain stopper being gold mounted.(41, *right*) The bottle in the form of an olive is made of two enamelled plaques, on which flowers in yellow and white are enclosed in a setting of silver with garnets and rhinestones. Its clover leaf stopper is similarly jewelled.(42) Also likely to be French is the scent bottle in the form of a harp with blue stem and floral decoration and pastoral scenes. The foot opens to reveal a Watteauesque panel.(44) So too, is the bottle enamelled in bright pink and gold with miniature flowers on a white ground and having a gold cover to the stopper.(45) Two examples of Dresden workmanship are the biconical vase in two parts, the lower white, painted with roses, the upper part of brilliantly coloured flowers and foliage and having an enamel collar topped by a bird and an inscription 'Gage de mon amitié';(46) and the pear-shaped bottle richly decorated in Watteau style, the upper part with naturalistic pine-apple design, the stopper in the form of a stalk.(41, *left*) This may be contrasted with the heart-shaped bottle with a figure at the base. There are two rings for suspension, the arrow is in relief and the stopper is a flower fastened to the bottle with a tiny chain.(47)

Equally good porcelain scent bottles with metal mounts were being made at Chelsea during the period of Nicholas Sprimont, originally a silversmith. W. B. Honey is of opinion that the dark blue and claret coloured grounds of Chelsea wares were inspired by what had been done at Vincennes and he suggests that softer tones were adopted for the rococo style of the Chelsea figures than had been customary at Meissen.[1] Examples of Chelsea work(50) include delicate figurines, the heads serving as stoppers, and the three bottles in one, each a chicken with its engraved collar and chain in gold, with a fourth chicken at the base;(48) the bottle in tree form with the notary public writing a letter for the shy girl clinging to the flower-covered tree, the bottle having a gold stopper surmounted by flower petals.(49) Probably of Chelsea workmanship is the pear-shaped bottle in brilliant colours on which are figures apparently intent upon fishing: again the metal stopper takes the form of a dove or pigeon;(52) and the delicate tapering bottle with floral panels and a silver mount.(51)

ENAMELS

Workers in two centres in England, Battersea, London, and Bilston, Staffordshire, produced distinctive enamelled scent bottles. The Battersea Works at York House, started by S. T. Jansen, a one-time Lord Mayor of London, was shortlived, from 1753 to 1756. In its three years it could have furnished only a tithe of the pieces attributed to it. The Schreiber Collection in the Victoria and Albert Museum, London, has examples which show some of the characteristic colouring of true Battersea origin according to Honey which are crimson, bright blue and reddish brown. For a time Battersea employed two eminently skilled artists, S. F. Ravenet and Robert Hancock, both of whom used French designs for their pieces. An example of Battersea work is seen in the hexagonally-based bottle having flowers on a blue ground and landscapes in reserved panels, the metal stopper in the form of a dove.(41)

The first recorded enamellers in Bilston and the area round about it, including Birmingham, date from about 1750. In that district the making of enamelled snuff boxes and cases for scent bottles went on from the middle of the eighteenth century to the end of the nineteenth, though the

---

[1] Honey, W. B., *The Art of the Potter*, London, 1946, 84-5.

work coarsened during the latter period. The best period for collectors is the twenty years up to 1770.

The Bilston enamellers were first of all toy makers, for which they were accustomed to use copper-zinc alloys, decorating the toys with chasing, engraving or turning, and embellishing them with tortoiseshell, agate and so on. They began to use enamel as a variant and this new kind of decoration, once launched, gave rise to an enormous output, master-minded by a few families whose history has been closely studied.[2] The decoration, enamel on copper, derived from engravings of the period or the fancy of the artists. The two vinaigrettes, one in the form of a basin with chain attachment and with floral motifs,(53) and the other, egg shaped, heavily enamelled on gilt and with its finial in pearls,(54) are unlikely to be of Bilston manufacture but the oval patch box of silver, engraved with the name of its intended owner, Amy Clarke,(64) may well be from this source. Tapered oval filigree patch boxes are not uncommon.

Wedgwood scent bottles are sufficiently rare to attract bidders in the sale rooms, especially if the bottles are in black basalt, with bronzed and gilt medallions and beaded or floral borders or in a blue jasper ware with olive and green medallions in a border of white florettes. These flattened oval bottles appear to have been made to a standard size of 7 to 8 cm. in height, the variation depending upon the size of the stopper.

ETUIS, PERFUME AND COSMETIC CASES

The habit of varying the kind of perfume worn from one hour or one day to another was one which perfumers encouraged their clients to cultivate. They were provided with small cases, perhaps no more than 10 cm. high, that would hold two, three or four tiny stoppered bottles. Often covered in shagreen, mostly green, white or grey, the perfume could be varied at will. The tiny bottles were filled from larger containers by using the small silver funnel which normally formed part of the contents of the case. The bottles were mostly of plain glass, white or occasionally in colour. It is exceptional to find a case with bottles in blue bearing delicate gilt

---

[2] Benton, Eric, 'The Bilston Enamellers', *Trans. Eng. Ceramic Circle*, 1970, vol. 7, pt. 3, 166–90. Benton points out that the first trade directory to include Bilston, 1770, notes four enamel box makers. During the previous twenty years several apprentices to snuff box makers and box painters had been recorded.

country figures in garden surroundings such as that illustrated, *c.* 1770, possibly decorated if not made in London.(56)

The French examples, a coffret of the last quarter of the eighteenth century, in tortoiseshell encrusted with gold, shows Italian country-scenes; the fitted interior includes a crystal bottle with funnel;(57) and in shagreen with four bottles and funnel; and in decorated porcelain with bottles and accessories.(60) A much larger case, of equal quality is the burr walnut toilet case made for Sophia, daughter of George III, to hold two diamond-cut bottles, each capped in silver with the initial 'S' engraved on it.(58) Fitted cosmetic cases of George III reign are rarely found complete: they are usually round and about 6 cm. in diameter, made in ivory or bone, sometimes with black edgings. These have moire silk linings and were originally fitted with a recessed mirror in the lid, a tiny maulstick with the head covered for applying the rouge, for which an ivory container was supplied, and a patch compartment.

PORCELAIN AND POTTERY COSMETIC JARS

The variety of French jars bearing the names of Paris perfumers has been referred to in Chapter 3.(11) English pots of the same period or even late seventeenth century, were either plain white or splashed with blue and mauve spots. They were usually bucket shape, about 3 cm. high, or on pedestals, and held a small quantity of a cosmetic cream or rouge paste.(59) Some of these pots bear the names of the perfumers and, when purchased, offer scope for enquiry into the history of the perfumers for whom they were originally made.(61, 62)

Nineteenth century

The sustained industrialization of the late eighteenth century was in-creased during the nineteenth, and inventiveness coupled with the fac-ilities of canal transport, better roads and later, the railways, brought raw materials to new factories and facilitated distribution to all parts of the British Isles. Glass workers, metal workers, potters and case makers alike shared in the demand for containers of all kinds, not least those required to keep pace with the needs of the new and growing middle class whose use of perfume, cosmetics and dentifrices rose rapidly. Staffordshire potteries maintained a steady supply of jars and pots for the cosmetic trade. In the present-day search for Victoriana, surviving examples of these pots attract many collectors.

COSMETIC JARS AND POT LIDS

With appreciation of the decorative value of cosmetic jars and pot lids, often framed in roundels, has come a literature in which all types and values are represented.[3] Rare examples, for instance some illustrations of bears, now fetch hundreds of pounds.(66) It was about the middle of the nineteenth century that makers of cosmetics, tooth pastes and salves saw the publicity advantage arising from using the newly-invented process of colour printing on flat or rounded surfaces and began to order lids printed in colour for preparations sold in covered earthenware pots.[4] Pots bearing printed labels or printed with black and white transfer designs had been on sale many years earlier. The manufacturers who could not afford the new coloured lids kept to the old style. Soon after colour printing became possible we find Patey & Co. of Lombard Street, London, supplying Genuine Bear's Grease in a lidded pot depicting a chained bear, in a lace-like border. About that time too, John Gosnell & Co., London, issued a Cherry Tooth Paste, patronized by the Queen (Victoria), with the portrait of a young lady in yellow with a blackish surround. Cherry Tooth Paste and Areca Nut Tooth Paste were two of the best liked varieties during the latter half of the nineteenth century, judging by the many examples of these lids offered. Rimmel, a London Perfumer, had a fine cherry design in red and white with lettering on a yellow band. Lids of Wood's Areca Nut Tooth Paste jars, originally sold with their contents for 6d and 1s are plentiful. Jars bearing the names of London makers of tooth paste, like Delescot and Hamet,(63) both in business during the last half of the eighteenth century, are rare. In 1781 Jacob Hamet, then dentist to Her Majesty Queen Caroline and the Princess Amelia, patented his Essence of Pearl and Pearl Dentifrice. Three years later it was being

---

[3] Clarke, H. G., *The Centenary Pot Lid Book*, London, 1949; *The Pictorial Pot Lid Book*, London, 1960; Ball, A., *The Price Guide to Pot-Lids and other Underglaze Colour Prints on Pottery*, Antique Collectors Club, Woodbridge, 1970; Hume, Audrey Noël, 'Nineteenth-Century Tooth Paste Pots, *Chemist & Druggist*, 1956, *165*, 618–19.

[4] Patent by Jesse Austin (J. & F. Pratt), 1847.

advertised as 'newly discovered' by W. Bayley of the Civet Cat in Cock-spur Street, London. The collector should look out for these and for other dentifrice pots bearing the word 'Opiate'. These 'opiates' contained no opium but were composed of honey, chalk, orris powder and carmine made into a paste with perfume essences and syrup.

Shaving creams went into the same type of lidded pot, a scarce example being the SEMPERUDIAN paste made by Wm. Dixon of Southampton. The use of square or rectangular pots was not common but specimens can be found now and then.

Cold cream, both white and tinted, was one of the most favoured cosmetics during the century and it is still on sale. The transfer decoration of the pots in which it was sold, black or grey, include the name of the seller or preparer. About 1880 green curved rectangular jars, with white edging made their appearance, looking like poor quality Wedgwood. They were used by several makers, among them Barrett who described himself as a patentee and whose 'ICY' cold cream jar pictured a young man pushing a maiden in a sleigh.

Decorated pots were in general use to the end of the century. Manufacturers then seized upon the advantages of issuing pastes and semi-solid cream preparations in collapsible tubes. Nevertheless many cosmetic makers have preferred to use pottery or opal glass pots of original design to enhance the distinction of their products.

While pots labelled 'bear's grease', 'cold cream' and 'dentifrice' are typical of those of the eighteenth and nineteenth centuries to be found in Britain, there were some unusual preparations on sale in France during the nineteenth century, the containers of which would add variety to a collection. Examples are 'Veritable Moelle de Boeuf' (ox marrow), on which oxen are depicted, and 'Creme de Limaçon', made from the snail and used as an emollient, the pot decorated with boldly coloured snails. These pots of good quality porcelain, with parchment covers tied with coloured ribbons to match the decoration, had replaced the old type of tin-glazed earthenware (delftware) and those with a mushroom cap and pedestal base, known to the French as 'godets'.

SCENT BOTTLES

A—Pottery

The potters shared in the manufacture of scent bottles, decorating them with portrait heads of the later Hanoverians and of the youthful Queen

Victoria. The Queen's head appeared on many pocket-watch-shaped bottles, usually in pale gold, the arms of the countries in the British Isles at the back. Some of these bottles bear the Worcester factory mark on the base. Wedgwood produced octagonal or round bottles in blue with applied designs in white; the bottles were the size of a pocket watch, the stopper taking the place of the stem winder. Disk shape bottles were also made in willow pattern design in pale blue. Spode bottles of melon shape or flattened oval, 5 cm. high, were marked 'SPODE—STONE CHINA' and were patterned with flower petals in yellow and brown. Egg-shaped bottles in appropriate sizes, coloured and stoppered to resemble the eggs of gulls, blackbirds and thrushes, came from Birmingham about 1870. Italian bottles of lava, 5 cm. high, were offered to tourists in southern Italy. Tooled to look like shagreen with a girdle of rosettes, and with gold or gilt covers to the stoppers, they sold readily. The fashion for these probably stimulated Italian mosaic workers during the mid-nineteenth century to produce bottles about 4.5 cm. high, in gold and coloured glass mosaic, decorated with the heads of the Pope or Garibaldi.

B.—Glass

During the past hundred years or so the profile of the glass bottle has become increasingly important to the designer seeking a distinctive style for a new perfume.(67) Should it be round, with sharp edges, bulb, pear or gourd shape or cut to give a prismatic appearance? Neck and stopper also had to be chosen with care to link up with the bottle design. Some of these problems had been resolved in the eighteenth century simply by gilding or enamelling. Another method was to encase the bottle in gold filigree, adding a chain or clip for wearing as part of the chatelain, a customary accessory of the period. One particularly fine example of filigree work is the stand in the form of a swinging cradle with compartments in the cradle itself to hold three leaf-capped glass bottles. A drawer in the wooden base of the cradle stand takes the bottles when not in use. When the perfume is needed, the bottles stand in the cradle, the caps are removed and the heavy perfume can then discharge into the room.(68)

During the Second Empire glass manufacturers in France produced scent bottles in opaline (milky) glass which they decorated with flowers, figures, animals or geometrical designs. Shape was important but the decoration had to please the eye.(74, 75) The same kind of glass was used for rouge pots, where porcelain was not preferred.(70) These cup-shaped pots, 3 to 4 cm. high, with flat covers, were either undecorated or simply bore the name of the maker of the cosmetic.(69) Larger cosmetic jars of the same material were provided with ormulu mounts and fluted covers, or if in simple form, with only slight patterns in contrasting colours.(69)

In 1819 Apsley Pellat took out a patent for the technique of producing cameos on glass scent bottles. These captured the popular fancy, and the Company's cut glass bottles with coloured heads representing a favourite figure of the time, the Prince Regent, George IV, William IV, Queen Adelaide and others, were widely sold. The bottles, about 10 cm. high, had different cuttings and the stoppers of some were decorated with figures.(76)

After the Great Exhibition of 1851 the country seems to have been faced with a large output of cut glass in two colours, sometimes heavily engraved, the colours chosen for vivid contrast. Bottles with a plain matt surface, for example, an under colour of Venetian red with floral design in white or yellow, attracted the perfumer's attention. Fanciful shapes and varied colours, like the duck head, pale blue over red, were made by Woodward of Stourbridge in the 1880s.(79b) More often the choice of shape was that of a pear or long oval, not more than 1 cm. thick and usually fluted or engraved. Miniature writhen blue glass bottles, attributed to Nailsea and made in the first quarter of the nineteenth century, were sold at fairs. Some had the year inscribed on them: all had fluted necks. To protect scent bottles when travelling, cases made of *cuir bouilli* (hardened and moulded leather) were made.

Moulded bottles, from 8 to 18 cm. long, of rectangular or square section, stoppered and with a narrow bore, were made in Germany and Italy during the nineteenth century. These seem to have been intended for expensive perfumes. Judging by the large number surviving, they were cheap to produce and must have been popular. They have three or four depressed or facetted sections on opposite or on all four sides, possibly useful as finger grips. Most of these bottles have gold leaf or enamelled designs, either running the whole length of the bottle or only in the depressed sections.(72) Only a few had chains attached. The bottles were sent out originally in decorated paper boxes.

One way in which a lover of perfumes could have a choice was to purchase a glass container in the form of a cross, each section of which was a separate scent bottle, capped with silver.(73) Another means of providing a larger selection for use in the home was adopted by the French during the Second Empire: this was to make heavy metal bottles about 10 cm. high, holding about 70 mils (3 oz.), with mock ormulu mounts and stoppers, each bottle having its own metal stand. On each panel of the square bottle, inset in the metal, was a coloured enamel representation of the Arc de Triomphe, the Palais de Justice or some other important Paris building.

During the mid-nineteenth century double-ended scent bottles of clear glass, one of the pair for perfume, the other possibly for smelling salts, often took the form of opera glasses. These could be folded over, end to end, for convenience in packing. An alternative form, in this case a double vinaigrette, is neatly capped to allow each half to be used at a time.(79a)

A completely new style bottle was demanded by Mlle Coco Chanel, the couturier, when she decided to introduce her Chanel perfumes in the 1920s. This, with its squared shoulders and well-cut stopper, first used for No. 5, attracted considerable attention. The artist, Sem, could not resist picturing the scene.(77)

PIQUÉ

This is the name given to a form of decoration of boxes and containers of all kinds made of tortoiseshell or other hard materials, the decoration being done in gold or silver in a pricked inlay design. Different names are applied to the particular style of inlay, whether done in small points, heavy points or definite shapes. Scent bottle cases, holding two or more tiny bottles, are often about 7 cm. high, of flattened oval shape. Many were made in tortoiseshell. The cases are mostly in small point inlay, in radiating patterns or clusters though they are (55) found in the three varieties. The best French examples are of the periods of Louis XIV and Louis XV but already in the seventeenth century similar decorative inlay work had been done in England. Many of the superior examples were made in the middle of the eighteenth century. Cases made at the end of that century reflect the designs of the Adams Brothers. Victorians liked the more heavily decorated styles. Mechanical means of piercing and inlaying materials were introduced during the last quarter of the nineteenth century. Piqué decoration was applied to bone, marble and shagreen and even to Sheffield plate.

PERFUME SPRAYS

These were widely used during the last half of the nineteenth century. The choice was between a spray operated by a spring piston or by a rubber bulb, emitting the perfume as a fine mist-like vapour. Similar kinds are in use today: the modern aerosol pack is unlikely to be filled with a fine perfume.

POWDER BOXES AND COMPACTS

Metal boxes, japanned or enamelled and decorated with flowers were the earliest produced in quantity from about 1850. Later machine finished compacts were in gilt or colour. Though most are round in shape for convenience in holding a powder puff, the tea-caddy shape was available for the dressing table.

SACHETS

Perfumers issued sachets filled with highly-scented powders as a means of keeping their names before the public. Enlivened with floral designs in colour and often with a calendar to invite their retention throughout the year, the sachets of the past century now take a place alongside the Valentine cards of the same period.

LABELS

A series of labels ranging over the past two centuries can give added enjoyment to the collector of scent bottles and antiques associated with perfume. From the middle of the eighteenth century French perfumers were using their own designed labels to add distinctiveness to the specialties and to reinforce their advertising. These labels were in a single tone of black and carried the name and address of the proprietor with a simple device. Once the rapid rise to fame of Napoleon I was assured a Pommade Napoleon label depicting him backed by the tricolour started a whole series of portrait labels.(80) Simple black labels were not to the liking of firms like Laugier who for his 'Eau de Montagnes Russes', on sale from 1814, used scenes of Russian life, snowy mountains, sleighs, Cossacks and pine trees. Distillers in Grasse contented themselves with depicting flowers or the equipment used for producing oils by distillation.

When colour printers could supply floral labels these were quickly adopted by the leading Paris Houses. Their fashion plate labels in colour for perfumes like Extrait de Bouquet and Fleurs d'Italie suggest a page from *Vogue*, had it then been current, but they had to compete with labels bearing life-like roses and carnations. Beginning with the Second Empire, Paris perfumers holding Court appointments brought out perfumes to please their royal patrons, the Emperor Napoleon III and the Empress Eugénie, using such labels as 'Parfum Favori de l'Impératrice', the elegant lady herself depicted in silken robe, a 'Bouquet Solferino', styled Parfum Impérial et Royal, with the Emperor and the victorious general of Solferino, both with moustaches and beards, and a 'Bouquet Exquis du Prince Impérial'. These were creations of Ed. Pinaud. Not to be outdone, Roger & Gallet had a 'Souvenir de la Cour' perfume and this and other portrait labels pictured ladies of the Court in charming décolleté. For rouge pots there was a series of delicate roundels which had to be trimmed by hand to fit the individual pots. Some of these labels were in relief and flowers like cyclamen or mimosa were commonly shown.

During the nineteenth century when the elaborate cut glass bottles were giving way to simpler but first-class designs, tiny labels bearing only the name of the perfume and its maker were used by most of the leading perfumers. The quality of the water-white glass and the colour of the perfume were considered all-important. To match the Art Nouveau and the French Art Deco bottles a completely new series of labels was designed by artists to ensure that the perfumers kept in line with the trend. Chemists in Britain, meanwhile, who were then supplying much of the perfume sold, contented themselves with plain or indifferently produced labels though the perfumery houses launched out into startling colours drawn in a free style. Throughout the whole period label designs have reflected changes in art fashions.(82)

PERFUME STAMPS

The practice instituted in Britain in 1786 of imposing a tax on perfumery and cosmetics to be paid by the affixing of revenue stamps to packages, though shortlived, was adopted in the late nineteenth century and during the present century by several countries, as widely spaced as Argentina, Panama, Portugal, Russia and the USA. There is now considerable interest in these stamps not only by specialists in philately but for the light they throw upon social history. The duty stamps of some countries, e.g. Portugal, were in use for only a few years and they have acquired a rarity value that appeals to collectors.(81)

7

Perfumers' and Perfumery Advertisements

Signs and Signboards

THE *Civet Cat* was by far the most favoured shop sign adopted by perfumers in the City of London and elsewhere from the time of the Great Fire of 1666. Most of the recorded signs are of the eighteenth century. By the middle of that century signboards and signs had become a nuisance and a danger to passers-by and in 1762 when streets had to be numbered the majority of the signs disappeared. For the most part only wall signs remained.

The Civet Cat was used by Francis Street, over against the Exeter Exchange, Strand, and by W. Bayley of Cockspur Street at the bottom of the Haymarket; the Civet Cat & Rose by D. Rigge of the perfumery warehouse in Cheapside;(84) the Civet Cat & the King's Arms by Wintle of Fleet Street (now Child's Bank); and the Civet Cat and Orange by Mr Rogers of Cheapside who sold Greek Water for venereal disease.

One Civet Cat sign remains in London, that over Barclay's Bank at the corner of Church Street and High Street, Kensington. 'YE CIVET CAT' was an old Inn in Kensington and when the bank took over the premises in 1920 a condition was imposed that the sign should be retained. (*Country Life*, 1965, pp. 401, 571, 624). The dark bronze or iron sign can be seen high up over the pavement.(83)

Other signs of perfumers included the Black Moor's Head in Exchange Alley; the Blue-Coat Boy, Cornhill, and the Blue-Coat Boy & Fan by sellers of the Royal Chemical Washball; the Red Ball & Acorn, Queen Street, Cheapside; the Green Ball, Bow Lane, Cheapside; and the Black Boy & Comb in Fleet Street. Mrs Giles, a milliner, of the Blue Ball by the Temple in Fleet Street, sold Washballs of a 'grateful and pleasant Scent, without the least Grain of Mercury and may be eaten for their Safety'.[1]

---

[1] Many of these signs were noted by F. G. Hilton Price in the *London Topographical Record*, London, 1904-5-6-7 under the heading 'Signs of Old London', vols. II to V.

Handbills, leaflets and cards

Most perfumers issued handbills, chiefly long lists of the various classes of goods they offered. These mostly follow a pattern though the order varied —powders, perfumed waters, essences, oils, soaps, washballs and pastes. Then came lists of sundries, hairpins, rollers, powder boxes, combs and brushes, tooth pastes and teeth instruments. These were followed by the perfumer's own specialties such as French Powder Engines for spraying the hair (Barnard's Old Perfume-Shop, kept by his daughter, G. Storer, 1696), Lip Salve of Tea Blossoms (D. Rigge), Italian Books full of Essences of the Choicest Odours, and Perfumed Garters and Sedan Garters (Lewis and David Bourgeois, 1777). Many of these bills were headed with trading devices.(85)

From 1830 the Paris proprietors of Eau de Cologne issued a series of cards portraying Jean Paul Féminis, the inventor, and his successors, Jean Marie Farina and Roger & Gallet. These called attention to its distribution 'avec profusion chez tous les peuples civilisés' and its acceptance by the Emperor, Napoleon I, and the principal Courts of Europe. Vourloud, Paris, issued a competing card shortly after his brevet of 1823.(78a)

Cards in colour as hand-outs up to 9 × 13 cm. were much in vogue in the USA during the last quarter of the nineteenth century. Using these, perfumes and soaps were well advertised, and Austin & Co. of Oswego went to the length of perfuming their cards to impress their Forest Flower Cologne upon likely customers. Book markers were also printed to ensure their retention.(88) This kind of card was used less in Britain than abroad, though E. W. Falk of 1 Vine Street, America Square, London, had cards for his Imperial Pastilles for fumigating rooms.

Towards the end of the nineteenth century designs were in the Art Nouveau style with flowing curves, a style illustrated by the Poudre d'Iris de Florence, au Pilon d'Or,(87) Paris. The well known 'Bubbles' for Pear's Soap came in this century.(89) Showcards are so ephemeral that having served their temporary purpose they are quickly discarded. Few in use during the nineteenth century seem to have survived though some may have been used on screens and in scrap books. (78b, 86).

Advertisements

Though advertisements of books and of medicines were published during

1652 in *A Perfect Diurnal* and were continued spasmodically thereafter, it was almost a century before it was regarded as good form to advertise one's wares in the public press. The *London Gazette* of 14–18 June 1666 told its readers that advertisements of 'Books, medicines and other things (were) not properly the business of a Paper of Intelligence'. Nevertheless the respectable *Gazette* continued to accept such advertisements for almost a century after its announcement.

In 1660–1 dentrifice manufacturers, using the *Public Intelligencer*, started to make known their 'Dentrifices to scour and cleanse the Teeth' and they continued throughout the next century and a half up to 1800, bringing before the public such items as Indian Dentiffick Roots and an Acidulous Alkaline Dentifrice.

By 1697 the perfumers had begun. In the *Post Boy* of 15–17 January, John Lawrence, an Italian perfumer, announcing his removal to the Strand, London, states he has received '. . . a parcel of the very finest Perfumes, and Spirits of Jessamy (Jasmine) and Orange and Spirits of Brigamot (Bergamot), and Pomatiums, Jessamy-Chocolet . . . and other Odors . . .'. *Defoe's Review* of 12 August 1704, offers 'The Royal Essence for the Hair . . . an unparallelled fine Scent for the Pocket and perfumes Hankerchiefs, etc.' In the same year 'The Golden Odoriferous Essence of Johannes Rosarious, M.D. & Philochym,' was recommended by a periwig maker.

At the beginning of the eighteenth century hair dyes were widely advertised. Lockton, at the Griffin toy shop, sold a 'Chymical Liquor' to turn hair, whether red, grey or any other disagreeable colour, into brown or black 'that neither time nor weather could alter'. Even the *Spectator* did not disdain the revenue from the promoter of the 'Famous Bavarian Red Liquor' which gave a delightful blushing colour to the cheeks: the use of which could not be perceived to be artificial by the nearest friend. In 1777 Sharp, a ladies' hairdresser of the Three Lilies in New Bond Street, recommended his Elastic Cushions for the hair, of a peculiar elegance and lightness, 'requiring fewer pins and less trouble than anything else'. He supplied beautiful hair for chignons. John Pyke of Cheapside offered ladies' Toupees, light in weight and needing no knot or bow of hair to make them complete. The public who required bear's grease as a hair pomade were periodically notified through the press of the killing of bears for that purpose and were invited to see this done. A 'Gentlewoman' at the Red Ball and Acorn in Queen Street, Cheapside, who in 1721 was selling an incomparable Wash to beautify the Face from half a crown to £5 a bottle, very obligingly kept a light hanging in the entry for her night customers.

Although there were importations of foreign flower oils in bulk—jars of Oil of Rosemary and Oil of Bays being sold by auction 'By the Candle' at the Marine Coffee House in Birchin Lane, London, in 1744—it was not until 1799 that advertisements for imported perfumery became general. Pommade de Grasse appeared in 1777 and the Bloom of Ninon was available in 1784, probably an imitation of the Parisian 'Eau de Ninon de l'Enclos' introduced a century before.

By this time the ethical views about publicity expressed in the 1660s had changed: in 1782 the proprietors of Speediman's Stomach Pills stated 'It has become the necessary custom of the times that medicines even of the most approved effects should be regularly held up to the public'. It was then, according to the late Lord Rosebery, that 'the age of advertisement' was begun. Soap had been advertised by the indirect method in 1679 by Timothy Cox in *The True Domestick Intelligence* of 2 December— 'Whereas one *Deval* has spread abroad a report in commendation of his *Sope*; be pleased to take notice, that as touching the goodness and substantialness of *Sope*, either White or Coloured, there cannot be better in the World than what is made by Timothy Cox . . . whose proper employment it is, and not *the Scale-makers*'.

Vinaigrettes have been described in Chapter 3. An advertisement in the *Post Boy* of 16–18 April 1700 suggests that a kind of smelling salts was then coming on the market—'The Volatile Aromatic Salt, for the Pocket, of a most Fragrant . . . scent, being wholly free from Musk, Civet, or any thing offensive to the Brain'. In 1785 Dalmahoy of London, a chemist to Her Majesty, advertised his 'Curious Smelling Bottle' in French as the Bouteille de Senteur. About the year 1820, A. Rowland & Son, London, almost swamped the country with their bills for Macassar Oil and Kalydor for the Complexion. Threefold leaflets in colour portrayed ladies with hair to their ankles. Kalydor arrested the advance of time and old age and though 'Powerful in Effect it was mild of Influence'. The end of the nineteenth century brought numerous advertisers into play. Beetham's of Cheltenham tried to keep in line with those who resorted to rhyme: 'But now in Old Sol's burning rays She sweetly dares to slumber, For Beetham puts her all to rights With Glyc'rine and Cucumber'.

Advertising gimmicks are now commonplace but that adopted by John Gosnell & Co., perfumers, London, in 1893 was, to say the least, out of the ordinary. This was long before skywriting was possible. Gosnells had a balloon made in the shape of a bottle of their 'Cherry Blossom' perfume. On the side of the balloon was a facsimile label 40 ft wide and 30 ft high.

The cork and neck of the bottle stood 15 ft high beyond the shoulder. The whole was covered with a net which suspended a hoop and the balloon car below the bottle. The balloon was filled with gas at Sheffield and was flown by Griffith Brewer and Parker Hides. As Brewer relates in *Fiftytwo Years of Flying*, the experiment was successful, the balloon shot up fast and showers of leaflets advertising the perfume were dropped out like ballast. In all, Gosnells had three balloons made, one of which made passenger flights over Paris (Gosnells had a Paris branch); another was used for a time as a more or less stationary sky sign over London Bridge.[2]

Pottery and Glass Objects

In addition to the inscribed and decorated pots described in Chapters 3 and 7, some perfumery houses, in order to assist the retailers of their preparations, provided display objects that are now thought worth collecting. Examples of the white glazed pottery bear made for James Atkinson in the first quarter of the nineteenth century are now rarities— few specimens are known. There are two varieties, each about 40 cm. in length and about 20 cm. in height: a bear with solid paws on which is a glazed ribbon giving the name 'JAMES ATKINSONS BEARS GREASE' in black lettering across the body and '44 GERRARD STREET' in a glazed ribbon on the plinth below, the plinth made to imitate rocks and seaweed in blue and green;(16) and a bear with divided paws, with almost the same ribbon inscription but omitting the name JAMES, the address being painted directly on the plinth below and not on a ribbon. Alec Davis is of opinion these bears were made for Atkinson by Wood & Caldwell who were working as partners at Burslem, Staffordshire between 1790 and 1818.[3] Enoch Wood was the second son of Aaron Wood, a modeller and mould maker, whose brother Ralph made rustic figures like 'The Vicar & Moses'.

Examples of the pottery Lavender Water Group first issued by Yardley & Co., London, in 1913–14 also show slight differences. The word 'Dresden' in script which appears underneath the plinth of some specimens is missing from others. Some collectors have effaced the words 'YARDLEY's

---

[2] *Through the Fragrant Years—A History of the House of Gosnell, 1677–1947*, London, 1947.

[3] Davis, Alec, *Package and Print*, London, 1968.

Old English LAVENDER' from the shell enclosing them on the plinth. The colours of the figures are pleasing and the grouping attractive(15).

Though not issued by manufacturers to promote sales but rather as stock containers, the white flint glass-stoppered bottles holding from one to two pints of perfume and in use by many chemists during the first years of this century, may be mentioned. These bottles were labelled ESS. BOUQUET, JOCKEY CLUB, etc., in etched panels, shields or rectangles, some with the names of the contents engraved in the glass. These are less common than the usual chemists' bottles and they recall an age when purchasers of perfume were constant in their adherence to standard selections, long before the specialist perfumers had invented the names now so popular.

Perfumers' Trade Tokens

Most traders had to issue tokens of ¼d, ½d, or 1d, sometimes silver shillings, when there was a shortage of small change. This happened during three periods—early in the seventeenth century up to 1672 when the Mint under the direction of Charles II made a large issue of farthings and halfpennies, though tokens continued to be used in the provinces because it was profitable to melt down the official coins; the first half of the eighteenth century because no copper coins were issued by the Mint until 1762-3 and 1771-3; and the late eighteenth century, during a period when the Mint was run inefficiently and tradesmen bought tokens in bulk from contractors. Silver tokens were suppressed by Parliament in 1813 and copper tokens in 1818. In addition to the trader's name and town or village, the tokens usually bore an emblem of his trade. Many hairdressers issued tokens but few perfumers are listed in the standard works. G. C. Williamson[4] records only one in the seventeenth century. This was issued by Nevell Harwar of New Cheapside, London, and bore on the Obverse: NEVELL. HARWAR. AT. YE CIVET(with a civet cat) and on the Reverse: IN. NEW. CHEAPSIDE=BAL & POWDER SHOP. The many distillers' tokens of the same century, mostly in Ireland, were presumably those of distillers of spirits and vinegars.

---

[4] Williamson, G. C., *Tradesmen's Tokens Issued in the Seventeenth Century in England, Wales and Ireland*, London, 1963 (Reprint), II, 678.

An eighteenth century ½d. token of Isaac Swainson of Middlesex shows a female figure dropping herbs into a still. This represented Hygeia preparing 'Velno's Vegetable Syrup' and was partly an advertisement for this nostrum. This token, with a minor alteration was also issued in Ayrshire.[5] The only other token noted so far in any way relating to perfume was an eighteenth century token of Wm. Davidson, a chemist and druggist of Alnwick, Northumberland, who was also a stationer and printer, and whose tokens bore the words NOSTRUMS & PERFUMES.[6]

Cartoons and Caricatures

On the whole, caricaturists have found little for their brush or pen in the perfumery industry or in the extravagant use of perfume at some periods. (77) Styles of hairdressing and the use of hair powder have often lent themselves as subjects for the caustic comment of the artist. For example, a series by Gillray and others, some political, came out when the hair powder tax was imposed in 1795. This had followed a spate of drawings during the decade 1770–1780 based on the macaronic styles of elaborately swept-up hair adopted by both dandies and their ladies. The satires published by M. Darley, 39 Strand, London, from 1770 onwards portray figures of the *demi-monde*, but although many are of the Vauxhall Gardens type, wearing face patches, there is no mention of perfume as an adjunct to their attractions, though heavy make-up appears in many coloured drawings. In describing the illustrations to her book *A History of Make-up* (London, 1970), Maggie Angeloglou calls attention to portraits which clearly show the application of cosmetics, e.g. that of an Elizabethan Lady, late 16th century, in the Bodleian Library, Oxford.

The French satirist Henri Daumier turned his wit to most subjects: in his series *Croquis Parisiens* and *Robert Macaire* he used perfumery as a topic with which to tilt at the Establishment.

In a series of 'Personnages revétus des attributs de leur profession', an album depicting some eighty persons attired with the apparatus of their trades or professions, published before 1700 by Nicolas de Larmessin

---

[5] Atkins, James, *Traders' Tokens of the Eighteenth Century*, London, 1892, 138, 299.

[6] Listed in the *Catalogue of the Montague Guest Collection of Badges, Tokens and Passes*, British Museum, London, 1930, No. 1264.

(1640–*c.* 1725), the young perfumer wears a cassolette or fuming pot as his headdress, emitting clouds of smoke, with fans as epaulettes, a perfumed Spanish leather skin as a handkerchief, and carrying a tray of all sorts of essences, soaps and pomades, his coat hung with packages of pastilles, waters and powders. There have been similar attempts to portray persons wearing the utensils or wares associated with their occupations. In the nineteenth century, Bouchot of Paris, had a watercolour drawing of 'La Parfumeuse', a lady standing by a counter of bottles and jars, lavishly draped with a Spanish leather over a still, her skirt, her leg-of-mutton sleeves made of a sponge and a container filled with soap balls, and her headdress a pomade box.

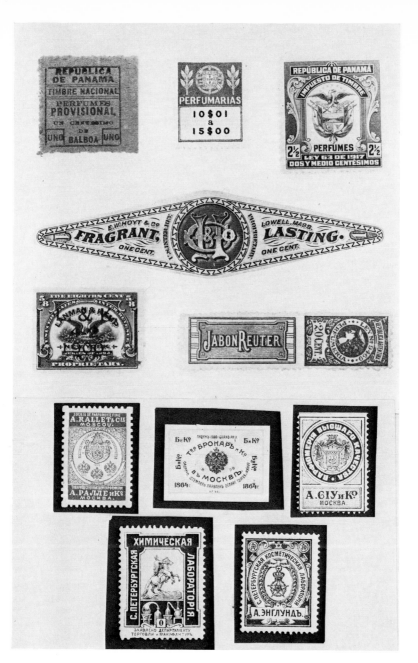

81. *REVENUE STAMPS & STAMP-LABELS FOR PERFUMES AND COSMETICS, 19TH &*
20TH CENTURIES
Panama, provisional, 1917; Portugal, 1924–6; Panama, regular issue, c. 1917.
U.S.A. E. W. Hoyt's German Cologne, 1877–82.
U.S.A. Lanman & Kemp, 1900; Argentina, Jabon Reuter, c. 1905. (George B. Griffenhagen Collection)
Russian stamp-labels of various manufacturers. (Collection of Emile Marcovitch, New York)

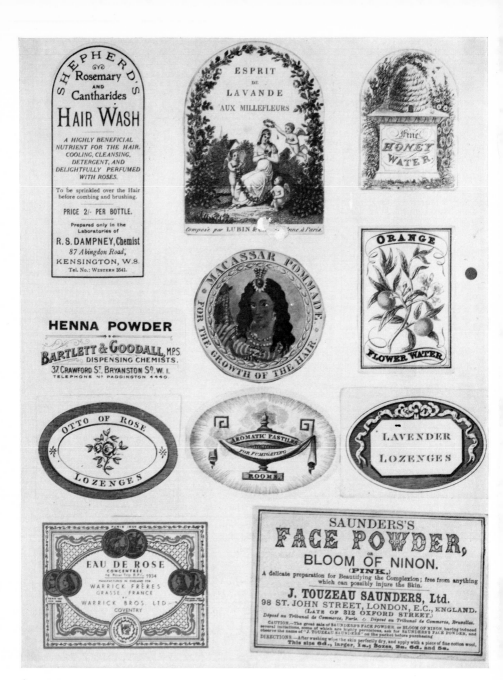

82. PERFUME LABELS, 19TH CENTURY
Those for Esprit de Lavande and Macassar Pommade are French, about 1850. The Face Powder label 'Bloom of Ninon' (bottom, right) recalls the special perfume named after Ninon de l'Enclos in the seventeenth century. (Private Collection)

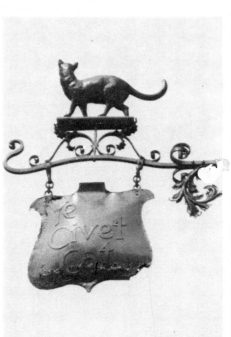
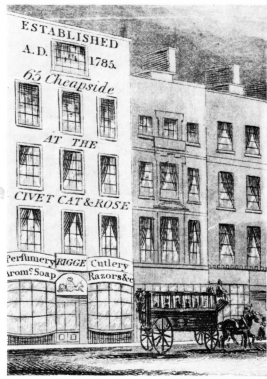

83. (above, left) THE CIVET CAT SIGN IN LONDON
Over Barclay's Bank at the corner of High Street and Church Street, Kensington. Formerly an Inn sign.
84. (above, right) RIGGE'S PERFUMERY WAREHOUSE, 65 CHEAPSIDE, LONDON, EARLY 19TH CENTURY
D. Rigge used 'The Civet Cat & Rose' as his trading sign and on his billheads. (Guildhall Museum, London)

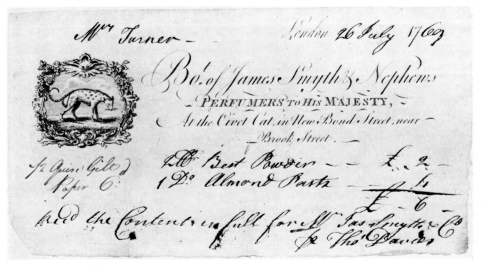

85. BILLHEAD, JAMES SMYTH & NEPHEWS, LONDON, 1769
At the Civet Cat in New Bond Street, near Brook Street. (Guildhall Museum, London)

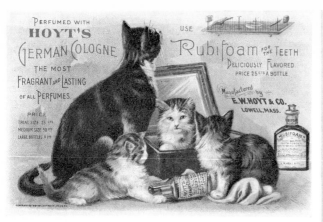

86 and 88. (left) ADVER-
TISING CARDS, U.S.A.,
LATE 19TH CENTURY

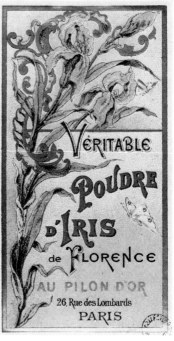

87. (above, right) SHOWCARD, POUDRE D'IRIS DE FLO-
RENCE, 19TH CENTURY
Au Pilon d'Or, Paris. (Bouvet Collection, Paris. Photo: Françoise
Foliot, Paris)
89. (below) SHOWCARD FOR PEAR'S SOAP, c. 1890
(One of the series 'The Signs & Sounds of Old London')

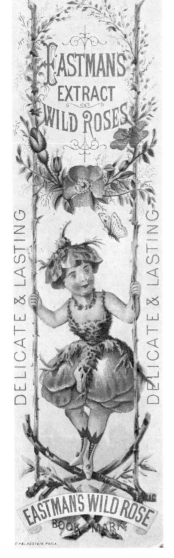

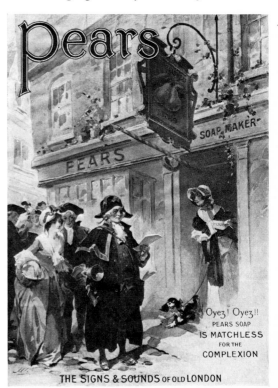

⟨ 8 ⟩

Some Special Uses of Perfume

Perfume and the Cult of Martys

THOUGH the Romans had strict laws forbidding interference in cemeteries, remains of Saints were often parted, even after cremation, and ashes, bones, and parts of sarcophaguses were eagerly sought. Once the cult of martyrs had begun in the fourth century AD in Milan, it spread widely to the Levant and to Egypt. Perfume and aromatic ointments were poured on the stone covers of the tombs in which the martyrs were buried. This became so general a practice that in many covers holes were purposely made to receive the perfume and ointments deposited by the faithful. It then became customary to bring phials or other receptacles to carry away some of the perfume or ointment deposited, as a reliquary to be revered. The invocation of martyrs came naturally to those who had paid their pious homage.[1]

2. Coronation Oil

The practice of anointing monarchs as a sign of divine favour was adopted in medieval times but for a limited number of rulers, for the Holy Roman Emperor, for the Kings of England, France, Jerusalem, Sicily, and by special Papal dispensation, for the Kings of Scotland. In England this practice has continued uninterruptedly. Up to the Reformation a special 'chrism', oil mixed with aromatic balsam, was used. Queen Elizabeth I had to be content with a simple oil which displeased her. At the coronation of James I the ceremony of anointing was omitted since this had

---

[1] Delahaye, Hippolyte, *Les Origines du Culte des Martyrs*, Brussels, 1933, 2nd. ed. 100, 117.

already taken place when he became James VI of Scotland. For the coronation of Charles I a special oil was devised by Sir Theodore Turquet de Mayerne, the King's chief physician who was also an able pharmacist. The ingredients included orange flower and jasmine oils in oil of benjamin, oil of roses and cinnamon, flowers of benzoin, ambergris, musk and civet. All these had to be mixed over gentle heat, spirit of rosemary being added to complete the preparation. At the Coronation Service the Oil is contained in an ampulla of gold, in the shape of an eagle. The Oil is poured from a silver gilt spoon, jewelled and enamelled, and which may date from the twelfth century. In the spacious days of George I the bill from the royal apothecaries for preparing the Oil came to £206 and a similar amount appeared in the accounts for George II.

By the time of the Coronation of Queen Victoria in 1837, the royal apothecaries had ceased to be practitioners of pharmacy and the Oil was prepared by Her Majesty's pharmaceutical chemist, Peter Squire. Subsequently it has been prepared by his successors, Squire & Sons of Oxford Street, London, and in turn by their successors, Savory & Moore of Bond Street. The Oil, the formula of which is secret, is amber coloured when freshly prepared and is said to possess a rich and peculiarly fragrant odour.

3. Incense

Reference has been made earlier to the practice of peoples like the Egyptians and the Hebrews of using incense in their religious rites. Among the many richly aromatic woods and gums for this purpose were myrrh, aloe wood, frankincense or opobalsam, benzoin and storax. For centuries the trade in almost all of these was in the hands of the Arabs. Strabo, c. 280 BC gave the 'happy land of the Sabaeans' as the source of many fragrant gums. Incense had its use as a purifier in churches when it was customary for the dead to be buried there.

Myrrh and frankincense, two of the aromatic gums, have continued to be used in incense into this century. A typical recipe for church use included these two gums, with benzoin, storax and cascarilla, nitre and sugar being added to ensure igniting the other components.[2] The Great Censer of St James of Compostela, northwest Spain, standing almost a

---

[2] Wootton, *op. cit. I*, 58.

metre in height and needing ten men to swing it to the roof of the huge cathedral, has its great pan of incense ignited with glowing charcoal to maintain a steady stream of sweet-smelling odours.

4. *Foods*

The use of perfumes in cooking has a long history. Pliny refers to the Roman taste for rose-flavoured dishes. Spices, probably first employed in the East where so many natural substances, seeds, balsams and cloves, were readily obtainable, helped to vary the ordinary foods making up the staple diet of the peoples. Today a score of varieties of curries add piquancy to continuous rice dishes. Spices, either whole or mixed, add both flavour and odour to dishes otherwise insipid or unpalatable. A whole repertory of flavours from natural and synthetic substances to please the housewife and the family is provided by the culinary specialist who needs the same kind of perception as the perfumer. The food specialist has to go further, he has to be sure that his additives are attractive to the eye and to the taste if he is to give the consumer complete satisfaction.

5. *Embalming*

The Egyptian practice of embalming has been noticed in Chapter 1. In Britain the duty of providing the spices, gums and perfumes necessary for this devolved upon apothecaries who on occasion had also to assist or supervise the operation for deceased monarchs, their queens, and at times nobles in attendance at Court. J. H. Moorman[3] has noted that during the fatal illness of Edward I at Lanercost Abbey in 1306–7 his medical advisers thought it prudent to have in reserve quantities of aloes, incense, myrrh and musk for the embalming of the King. The embalming of Queen Elinor, wife of Edward III, who died at Harby, Lincolnshire, on 28 November 1290, was carried out at the Gilbertine Priory of Lincoln; most likely the materials were supplied by her apothecary.

The cost of embalming a monarch was high: that for James I in 1625

---

[3] Moorman, J. H., *Eng. Hist. Records*, 1952, 67, 161–74.

was £282. 9s and only a little less for Charles II in 1685—£218. 8s. There is a full account of what was needed for Queen Mary, wife of William III, in 1694, when Dr Christian Harel had the task of embalming her body. The materials included rich gums and spices, damask powders and perfumes for the chambers and linen, the whole operation costing £300.

Comparable work was done by the Langeli family of pharmacists in Rome for over 200 years. They held the Pontifical pharmacy and with this went the duty of embalming each Pope at his decease. The pharmacy remained in their hands into this century. The last Pope for whom Louis Langeli's services in this manner were needed was Leo XIII who died in 1903.

6. *Aphrodisiacs*

Many perfumes have been devised to excite the attractiveness of the sexes and at times it has been the vogue to add so-called aphrodisiacs to accentuate this and by skilful advertising, to increase sales. A special perfume, quoted by Lémery, the celebrated French chemist in the eighteenth century, and known as 'l'Elixir de Magnaminité', was said to increase venery. It had as its principal ingredients muscade, satyrion (from an orchid with a goat-like scent), cardamoms, animal substances, musk and ambergris. It was almost guaranteed as a cure for impotency.[4] In *Aphrodisiacs and Love Stimulants* by John Davenport (re-issued, London, 1965), ambergris is reported to produce a marked acceleration of the pulse and a quickening of the senses, and the use of musk by Madame du Barry in her relations with Louis XV strengthened a disposition to cheerfulness and venery. In the early part of the present century patchouli perfume was reputed to be powerfully attractive to the male and in consequence was much used in London's West End.

---

[4] Paressant, Charles, *L'Etude des Rapports entre la Pharmacie et la Parfumerie*, (Thèse Doctorat de l'université), Nantes, 1957, p. 41.

Select Bibliography

Allhusen, Dorothy *Book of Scents and Dishes*, London, 1926.

Angeloglou, Maggie *A History of Make-up*, London, 1970.

Arctander, Steffan *Perfume and Flavour Materials of Natural Origin*, Elizabeth, New Jersey, USA, 1960.

A Rich Closet of Physical Secrets, London, 1652. Printed by Gartrude Dawson.

Atkins, James *Traders' Tokens of the Eighteenth Century*, London, 1892.

Ball, A. *The Price Guide to Pot-Lids and Other Underglaze Colour Prints on Pottery*, Woodbridge, 1970.

Barbe, Simon *Le Parfumeur Royal*, Paris, 1699.

Bear, I. J. & Thomas, R. G. 'The Nature of Argillaceous Odour and Genesis of Petrichor', *Nature*, 1964, *201*, 993; *Geochimica et Cosmochimica*, 1966, *30*, 869–79.

Bedford, John *All Kinds of Small Boxes*, London, 1964.

Bennet, H. *The New Cosmetic Formulary*, New York, 1970.

Benton, Eric 'The Bilston Enamellers', *Trans. Eng. Ceramic Circle*, 1970, 7, pt. 3.

Blackman, R. J. *Life of Sir Edward Wild*, London, 1935.

Blaizot, Pierre *Parfums et Parfumeurs*, Paris, 1946.

Bovill, E. W. 'Musk & Amber', *Notes & Queries*, 1953, *CXCVIII*. (Reprint)

Catalogue of the Montague Guest Collection of Badges, Tokens & Passes, London, 1930.

Clarke, H. G. *The Centenary Pot Lid Book*, London, 1949.

   The Pictorial Pot Lid Book, London, 1960.

Davenport, John *Aphrodisiacs and Love Stimulants*, London, 1965. (Re-issue)

Davis, Alec *Package & Print*, London, 1968.

Davis, W. J. *Nineteenth Century Token Coinage*, London, 1904.

Debay, Auguste *Les Parfums et les Fleurs*, Paris, 1846.

Delahaye, Hippolyte *Les Origines du Culte des Martyrs*, Brussels, 1933.

Dennis, R. *English Glass*, London, 1967.

'Eau de Cologne', *Chemist & Druggist*, London, 1875, *17*, 172–6.

Flückiger, F. A. & Hanbury, Daniel *Pharmacographia*, London, 1874.

Foster, Kate *Scent Bottles*, London, 1966.

Hibbott, H. W. *Handbook of Cosmetic Science*, London, 1963.

Hilton Price, F. G. 'Signs of Old London', *London Topographical Record*, London, 1904–7, vols. II to V.

Holmyard, E. J. *Alchemy*, Harmondsworth, 1957.

Honey, W. B. *The Art of the Potter*, London, 1946.

Irissou, L. 'Sur l'Origine de l'Eau de Cologne', *Rev. d'Hist. de la Pharmacie*, Paris, 1952, 262.

La France et Ses Parfums, Paris, 1960–70. A Bi-monthly Review. Various contributors.

La Parfumerie Française et l'Art dans la Presentation, Paris, 1925.

Latham, R. & Matthews, W. *The Diary of Samuel Pepys*, London, 1970, vol. I.

Launert, Edmund 'Scent & Scent Bottles', *Collector's Guide*, London, Aug. & Sept. 1971.

Lémery, Nicolas *Pharmacopée Universelle*, Paris, 1690.

Letters & Papers of Henry VIII, London, *XXI*, pt. 2.

Lillie's British Perfumer, ed. C. Mackenzie. London, 1822, 2nd ed.

Liste du Corps des Marchands—Gantiers—Poudriers—Perfumeurs . . . de Paris, Valleyre, Paris, n.d.

Manuscripts: British Museum: Cotton, Tiberius A vii (5); Royal 7c xvi; Sloane 5017*.

    Archives de la Seine, Paris: Faillites (Bankruptcies.)

Matthews, Leslie G. 'King John of France and the English Spicers', *Medical History*, 1961, *V.*

Mead, Richard *A Short Discourse concerning pestilential contagion . . .*, London, 1720.

Moncrieff, C. W. *The Chemical Senses*, London, 1967.

Myers, A. R. *The Household of Edward IV*, Manchester Univ. Press, 1959.

Norton, Thomas *The Ordinall of Alchemy*, London, 1928. (Facsimile)

Oliver, Raymond *The French at Table*, London, 1967.

Owen, R. *The Practice of Perfumery*, London, 1870.

Paressant, Charles *L'Etude des Rapports entre la Pharmacie et la Parfumerie*, Nantes, 1957.

Piesse, Septimus *Des Odeurs des Parfums*, Paris, 1877, 2nd. ed.

    Histoire des Parfums, Paris, 1905.

Pepys, S. *Private Correspondence & Misc. Papers, 1679–1703*, ed. J. R. Tanner, London, 1926.

Poucher, W. A. *Perfumes, Cosmetics & Soaps*, London, 1941, 3 vols.

Privy Purse Expenses of Henry VIII, 1529–32, ed. N. H. Nicolas. London, 1827.

Privy Purse Expenses of Princess Mary, ed. F. Madden, London, 1831.

'Queen Elizabeth's Perfume', *Pharm. Journal*, 1960, *185*, 502.

Rimmel, Eugène *The Book of Perfumes*, London, 1865.

Sagarin, E. *The Science and Art of Perfumery*, New York, 1945.

Salmon, W. *Pharmacopoeia Londinensis*, London, 1691, 4th ed.

Savage, George *Glass*, London, 1965.

Tanner, E. S. *May It Please Your Lordship*, London, 1971.

Thompson, C. J. S. *The Mystery & Lure of Perfume*, London, 1927.

Trease, G. E. 'The Spicers and Apothecaries of the Royal Households . . ., Hen. III, Ed. I, Ed. II.' *Nottingham Medieval Studies*, 1959, III.

Williams, Neville, J. *Powder & Paint, Elizabeth I to Elizabeth II*, London, 1957.

Williams-Wood, Cyril, *Staffordshire Pot Lids and Their Potters*, London, 1972.

Williamson, G. C. *Tradesmen's Tokens in the Seventeenth Century . . .*, London, 1963. (Reprint)

Wootton, A. C. *Chronicles of Pharmacy*, London, 1910.

Collections of Antiques of Perfume

London:	The British Museum, Great Russell Street, W.C.1.
	The London Museum, Kensington Palace, W.8.
	Victoria & Albert Museum, South Kensington, S.W.7.
	The Wellcome Institute of the History of Medicine, 183 Euston Road, N.W.1.
Birmingham:	City Museum & Art Gallery, Congreve Street.
Brighton:	Art Gallery & Museum, Church Street.
Bristol:	Blaise Castle Folk Museum, Henbury.
Cardiff:	The Welsh Folk Museum, St. Fagan's.
Derby:	Museum & Art Gallery, Strand.
France:	Ed. Pinaud (Laboratoires France-Parfum), 6 rue Champs, Asnières sur Seine, 92 Hauts-de-Seine.
	Givaudan France, 44 Boulevard du Parc, 92 Neuilly sur Seine.
	Guerlain, 25 rue Louis-Ulbach, Courbevoie, 92 Hauts-de-Seine.
	Musée des Arts Decoratifs, rue de Rivoli, Paris.
	Musée Fragonard, Grasse, Alpes Maritimes.
USA	Metropolitan Museum, New York.
	Houbigant Inc., Ridgefield, New Jersey.

Index

Numbers in Italic indicate Plate numbers